T0215341

Psychiatric Mental Health Assessment and Diagnosis of Adults for Advanced Practice Mental Health Nurses

This text provides a comprehensive and evidence-based introduction to psychiatric mental health assessment and diagnosis in advanced nursing practice.

Taking a clinical, case-based approach, this textbook is designed to support graduate nursing students who are studying psychiatric mental health nursing as they develop their reasoning and decision-making skills. It presents:

- Therapeutic communication and psychiatric interviewing techniques, alongside basic psychiatric terminologies.
- The major psychiatric diagnoses, drawing on the DSM-5.
- A step-by-step guide to conducting a comprehensive psychiatric mental health assessment.
- Case examples demonstrating assessment across major psychopathologies.
- Good practice for conducting mental health evaluations.

This is an essential text for all those undertaking psychiatric mental health nurse practitioner programs and a valuable reference for advanced practice nurses in clinical practice.

Kunsook S. Bernstein is Professor Emerita at Hunter College School of Nursing, City University of New York, where she taught advanced psychiatric nurse practitioner students and coordinated the psychiatric mental health nurse practitioner program. Her primary area of research is Asian American immigrants' mental health and healthcare disparities.

Robert Kaplan is Advanced Senior Lecturer and Co-Principal Investigator of the Writing Research Lab in the Program in Writing and Rhetoric at Stony Brook University, State University of New York. He teaches research writing to advanced undergraduate STEM students and is a science editor for public health researchers.

Psychiatric Mental Health Assessment and Diagnosis of Adults for Advanced Practice Mental Health Nurses

Kunsook S. Bernstein and Robert Kaplan

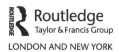

LONDON AND NEW YORK

Cover image: © Getty Images

First published 2023
by Routledge
4 Park Square, Milton Park, Abingdon, Oxon OX14 4RN

and by Routledge
605 Third Avenue, New York, NY 10158

Routledge is an imprint of the Taylor & Francis Group, an informa business

British Library Cataloguing-in-Publication Data
A catalogue record for this book is available from the British Library

Library of Congress Cataloging-in-Publication Data
A catalog record has been requested for this book

ISBN: 978-0-367-68455-6 (hbk)
ISBN: 978-0-367-68448-8 (pbk)
ISBN: 978-1-003-13759-7 (ebk)

DOI: 10.4324/9781003137597

Typeset in Times New Roman
By Deanta Global Publishing Services, Chennai, India

Dedicated to my husband, Steven, and to my mother,
Bong-Suk Koo, to my children, Joseph and Beth, and to my
grandchildren, Catherine, Peter, and Jacob
-Kunsook S. Bernstein

Dedicated to my parents, Harold and Lore W. Kaplan
-Robert Kaplan

Contents

Figures

Tables

Boxes

Introduction

Advanced psychiatric mental health nursing (APMHN) emerged as a graduate-level nursing specialization in the late 1950s, after the passage of the National Mental Health Act of 1946 and the creation of the National Institute of Mental Health in 1949, which has led to many advancements in mental health evaluation and treatment. While initially APMHNs were trained to practice autonomously, the degree has also evolved to prepare them to assess mental health problems, diagnose psychiatric disorders, and provide treatment independently. Concurrently, psychiatric treatment itself has shifted in its understanding of mental health disorders, from a psychodynamic basis to one that incorporates neurobiology, with the concomitant development of efficacious psychotropic medications. With the advancement of psychopharmacology, the role of the APMHN has further evolved to encompass the expanding biopsychosocial perspective, and the competencies required to practice have kept congruent with the emerging science. Consequently, many psychiatric mental health graduate nursing programs have modified their curricula to include greater emphasis on comprehensive mental and physical health problems, and on the professional competencies necessary for prescriptive authority (American Nurses Association, 2014).

This book is designed to assist APMHN students and early-career APMHNs to advance their competencies by explaining and demonstrating the steps required to conduct a comprehensive psychiatric mental health assessment, as well as to formulate the initial diagnosis of adults with psychiatric disorders, both of which are critical to the role of the APMHN. The book takes an incremental approach to guide its readers through this entire process of mental health assessment and diagnosis, but it does not focus on the treatment that would follow.

Fundamental to nursing philosophy is caring. Consequently, Chapter 1 explores the principles and guidelines of therapeutic interviewing, as it is through therapeutic communication that APMHNs demonstrate their understanding of their clients. The chapters that follow examine more specific applications of assessment and diagnosis to different mental health situations. Chapter 2 presents case-based differential diagnostic mental health evaluations and the neurobiology of mental illness, as to effectively prescribe medications to treat clients with mental illness it is essential that APMHNs be competent and knowledgeable about the neurobiological basis of mental disorders upon which psychopharmacology is based. In

DOI: 10.4324/9781003137597-1

fact, a separate course on psychopharmacology should be considered as part of the academic degree program; if one is not available, APMHNs should master the equivalent, whether or not it is required by each state's regulatory system. Chapter 3 provides practice guidelines for the assessment of high-risk behaviors, and Chapter 4 provides practice guidelines for cultural assessments.

Reference

American Nurses Association. (2014). *Scope and standard of psychiatric-mental health practice* (2nd ed.). American Nurses Association. ISBN: 978155810555

1 Therapeutic Interviewing and Mental Health Evaluation of Adults

Section 1: Principles of Therapeutic Interviewing

Therapeutic interviewing is the craft by which the advanced psychiatric mental health nurse (APMHN) attempts to clearly understand their clients. It can be an instrument of healing for individuals who are in both physical and psychological need, and therefore is an essential skill for APMHNs to learn and apply. It involves the use of verbal and nonverbal messages during the interview by tailoring the nurse's verbal skills to suit the unique physical and emotional needs of the client, as they are revealed. The aim is to establish a professional therapeutic nurse–client relationship that engages the client with the healing process. Consequently, the role of the APMHN, especially when interviewing a client for the initial psychiatric evaluation, goes beyond simply information gathering.

In this section of the chapter, the underlying principles of therapeutic interviewing are discussed. These principles, which may determine whether an initial interview fails or succeeds, are not rigid; instead, they provide flexible guidelines, discussed in the next section, within a structured framework that enable the interviewer to create a warm and safe atmosphere appropriate to the circumstances. The first encounter with the mental health clinician can be the beginning of the healing process for many clients seeking mental health services. Therefore, engaging in therapeutic interviewing while collecting pertinent clinical data, such as physical, mental, and emotional status, and conducting needs assessments is an art, and one necessary for the APMHN to be masterful in, to effectively promote their clients' healing.

Each interview may vary depending on the purpose, location, time allocation, and other circumstances. For example, an APMHN may interview a client who is scheduled for their initial psychiatric assessment and treatment at an allocated time in an outpatient clinic, or they may be assessing and interviewing a client in the emergency room for a psychiatric crisis. At other times, an APMHN may be called to evaluate a client in a general hospital or long-term care facility on a consultative basis, or they may work regularly in a psychiatric hospital conducting daily assessments and longer-term treatments of assigned clients. Yet, regardless of the context, to provide an effective interview during the psychiatric mental health assessment, an APMHN must have a broad sense of the assessment goals.

DOI: 10.4324/9781003137597-2

These goals will be explained in more detail in the Case Exemplar section of this chapter, but are presented briefly here for the reader to have a broad understanding of interview dynamics, as delineated by Shea (1998a), even though the different contexts within which an interview may occur, as noted above, may lead to certain goals being more important or more achievable than others in any particular interview or interview setting:

1. To establish a sound engagement of the client in a therapeutic alliance.
2. To collect a valid database.
3. To develop an evolving and compassionate understanding of the client.
4. To develop an assessment from which a tentative diagnosis can be made.
5. To develop an appropriate disposition and treatment plan.
6. To effect some decrease of anxiety in the client.
7. To instill hope and ensure that the client will return for the next appointment.

In addition, the APMHN must also have an awareness of the characteristics of a successful therapeutic relationship between clinician and client, whether that relationship consists of a single meeting or a series of meetings. Johnson and Vanderhoef (2016) defined those characteristics as genuine, empathetic, authentic, respectful, nonjudgmental, accepting, and maintaining professional boundaries. Ultimately, then, to formulate a mental health assessment and diagnosis through a skillful interview, the APMHN needs to be clear about the assessment goals, knowledgeable about the characteristics of therapeutic communication techniques, and cognizant of psychiatric terminology.

This section uses a case scenario to explore the core issues challenging APMHNs during mental health assessments. Based on the principles of therapeutic communication to interview clients with psychiatric disorders, the focus here is on the interactional process whereby APMHNs use commonly known therapeutic communication techniques, noted in Table 1.1, to build rapport with each client, while formulating a comprehensive mental health assessment, which leads to diagnosis. Finally, the chapter concludes with a glossary of common psychiatric terminology with which the APMHN must be familiar to write the formal assessment.

As the clinical interview constitutes an interactive relationship between a clinician and client, formulating a structure for it benefits both parties by creating a naturally occurring flow that allows the clinician to focus on guiding the interview in an efficient manner (Shea, 1998). This structure is highlighted in this section through three phases: (1) engagement, (2) valid data collection, and (3) closing of the interview. It is important to note that these phases do not always form a distinct progression; rather, the clinician can go back and forth between them as deemed necessary, based upon cues from the client, to successfully establish a rapport and to gather the necessary information.

The clinical case scenario presented below weaves between each phase by using therapeutic communication techniques with clear interview goals to begin to establish the characteristics of a therapeutic relationship, while collecting

Table 1.1 Therapeutic Communication Techniques and Examples

Technique	Example
Accepting	"What you said makes sense." Nodding.
Broad openings	"Is there anything you would like to talk about?"
Clarifying information	"I'm not sure I follow what you are trying to say."
Consensual validation	"Tell me whether my understanding of it agrees with yours."
Encouraging comparison	"Was it something like …?"
Encouraging expression	"Does this add to your stress?"
Exploring	"Tell me more about that."
Formulating a plan of action	"What would you do to channel your anger constructively?"
General leads	"Go on," "And then?"
Making observations	"You seem to be tense."
Offering self	"I will stay with you for a while."
Placing event in time or sequence	"What seems to lead up to …?"
Restating	Client: "I can't sleep, staying up all night." Nurse: "You have difficulty sleeping."
Seeking information	"I would like to hear from you your perspective about how you have been feeling and what's been going on."
Silence	Nurse provides time for the client to put feelings into words, to regain composure, or to continue talking.

Source: Adapted from Belleza (2020).

pertinent data to formulate a diagnosis of a mental disorder, ending with a documentation of a mental health evaluation.

Phase 1: Engagement

Therapeutic engagement is an interpersonal process in which a clinician aims to develop a particular type of personal relationship with the client in the first, and potentially only, session. Its purposes include assessing the client, developing a shared understanding of the contents of the discussion, and planning how to manage the client's experience of the interview. Engagement skills are then further used to develop a therapeutic relationship (Walker, 2014). As the initial contact for psychiatric evaluation can be highly anxiety producing for clients, the goal of the interviewer during this phase is relatively simple: decrease the client's anxiety and establish a sound engagement of the client in a therapeutic alliance using the therapeutic skills of genuineness, acceptance, and empathy. The client will form an initial impression of the APMHN and of the therapeutic encounter based on the APMHN's attitude, mood, and verbal and nonverbal presentations during this phase; therefore, the APMHN should be aware of their own comfort in interacting with the client, and be mindful of any triggers evoking either positive or negative emotional reactions.

The following is an example of the engagement phase during the client–APMHN initial psychiatric evaluation interview scenario, accompanied by an analysis.

The APMHN is working in a mental health outpatient clinic, and a new client is in the waiting room, scheduled for an initial psychiatric evaluation. Following clinic policy, the APMHN walks to the waiting room, greets the client, and the two walk back to the APHMN's office. While in the waiting room, the client completed a personal demographic information form (name, sex, age, referral source, insurance information, contact person, etc.), which they give to the clinician.

APMHN: (smiling warmly and spontaneously) Hi, my name is Peter Smith. I am a psychiatric nurse practitioner, and you have an appointment with me today for evaluation. (Upon arrival to the office.) Please have a seat and make yourself comfortable (the APMHN waits until the client sits down before sitting down, as a sign of courteousness).

Comments: This is a simple and common verbal introduction scenario of the engagement process. However, the APMHN's body language, gestures, and tone of voice give a first impression to the client as to whether or not the clinician is genuine and respectful.

Client: Thank you (avoiding eye contact and looking down to the floor).
APMHN: (Observing the client's body language and facial expression, asks a question in a soft tone of voice.) Do you have any preference as to how I should call you? Is it "Ms. Larson" or "Jane" or something else?

Comments: By acknowledging the client's cultural background and personal preference, this question allows the client to feel respected and empowered.

Client: Call me "Jane" (still not making eye contact).
APMHN: OK, Jane, since this is our first meeting, maybe you can tell me about yourself and what brought you here today?

Comments: This broad opening question guides the client to share personal matters and to determine which ones to share (seeking information). It is a commonly used phrase which turns the interview over to the client.

Client: My family thinks I am depressed and need to see someone.
APMHN: I see. … What do you think? I would like to hear from you about your perspective as to how you have been feeling and what's going on.

Comments: The APMHN encourages the client to express and elaborate on her feelings and thoughts in her own words.

Client: I don't know (pause). I guess I have been down for a while since I broke up with my boyfriend … (hesitant tone).
APMHN: Go on (said gently, leading the client to continue).

Comments: The APMHN's observation of the client's behaviors (avoiding eye contact, short sentence answers, and hesitation to talk) indicates that the client is reluctant to engage in the conversation. Therefore, the APMHN is using gentle leading to give the client room to engage at her own pace.

Client: Things have been rough since then. … Even though I am the one who broke up with him, I miss him, but the thought of getting back together makes me sick. So I don't know what to do and I did not want to say anything to my mother but she knew something was not right.

APMHN: (Silence, while allowing the client to continue.)

Comments: Since the client is slowly but slightly more engaged in sharing her story, silence is appropriate for the APMHN. At the same time, the APMHN assesses the initial mental health status of the client:

- Reason that the client is presenting for evaluation: *Difficulty coping following the break-up with the boyfriend.*
- Psychiatric symptoms: *Anxiety manifested by feelings of helplessness and loneliness.*

The engagement phase, including the client's initial impression of the APMHN, represents the most critical arena for establishing rapport. In this case scenario, the APMHN applies therapeutic communication skills to establish a sound engagement with the client with the goal of creating a therapeutic alliance. Once the APMHN is aware of the client's core pains and needs, and sees signs of the client's readiness to engage in the interview, the APMHN should prepare to enter the valid data collection phase of mental health assessment by easing into gathering pertinent clinical information while skillfully engaging the client.

The next scenario continues the interview by demonstrating how the APMHN skillfully applies several therapeutic skills during the transition to Phase 2—the examination of the client's mental status and the collection of clinical data—to enable the client to feel more comfortable opening up.

Client: I know getting back with him is not good for me the way things were with him, but he has been in my mind 24/7 (24 hours a day and 7 days a week) since the break-up. I can't sleep or eat, and I'm crying frequently … (sobbing). It's hard for me to talk about it to anyone.

APMHN: (Offers her a tissue.) Sounds like it's difficult for you to talk about it, and you have been suffering all alone. I am glad that you are able to open yourself up now. When did you break up with him and what triggered the break-up?

Comments: Several therapeutic skills are applied here while assessing the client's presenting signs and symptoms:

- Restating and validating: "Sounds like it's difficult for you to talk about it, and you have been suffering all alone."

- Encouraging expression: "I am glad that you are able to open yourself up now."
- Seeking information: "When did you break up with him and what triggered the break-up?" This question gathers information about how long the client has been suffering and the nature of the trauma (as a result of the break-up).
- Clinical data: Tearful affect with sad mood, sleep and appetite disturbances, thoughts preoccupied with the break-up.

Client: *Well ... 6 months ago, I found out accidently that he was seeing my best friend for over a year behind my back (crying uncontrollably). I am sorry (wiping her tears).*

APMHN: It's ok, no need to apologize, if this is the first time you are talking about this, it can be very painful to rehash. But at least you are able to talk about it, which can be the beginning of healing. You mentioned earlier that you can't sleep or eat; would you share with me what other problems you have experienced since the episode, like how it has affected your mood, social life, work, self-image, things like that?

Comments: The APMHN makes an effort to create a supportive atmosphere by validating the client's feelings with positive reinforcement, which can be conducive to help the client feel safe enough to begin sharing freely. At the same time, the APMHN attempts to gather factual data about the client's thinking, feeling, and behavior.

Client: Initially, I was angry, so angry that I felt like literally jumping out of my skin. But I did not say anything to him other than breaking up with him. For a while, I felt numb, nothing mattered, I had a hard time concentrating at work and not talking to anyone ... (pause).

APMHN: Sounds like you have been through a lot. How are you feeling now?

Comments: Open-ended question leading the client to continue and focus her feelings at the present time.

Client: Well ... before I came here, I did not know what to expect, but talking about what happened is not as bad as I thought. ... You asked me how I feel now, I had a knot in my stomach while waiting in the waiting room, but it's gone ... strange ... Sorry, I am rambling.

APMHN: Glad to hear that you got rid of that knot in your stomach (smiling). You seem to be at ease talking about what you have been bottling up inside. Let me ask you some concrete questions and please let me know if any topic makes you feel uncomfortable. Starting with your sleep and appetite, how many hours do you sleep at night? And have you lost any weight?

Comments: The APMHN invests effort in creating an atmosphere that is optimally conducive for the client to feel safe to begin sharing her problems, and the client is able to wander freely to whatever topic naturally occurs. Once the client becomes more engaged, the APMHN focuses on content, gathering factual data, including risk factors like suicidality.

Phase 2: Valid Data Collection of Client's Mental Status

In this phase, a clinician conducts a mental health assessment while collecting valid client information to determine what content should be included in it. This is done by asking the client questions that elucidate what they mean by the terminology that they use. The clinician needs to elicit and record behavioral facts, not simply the client's self-assessment of their conditions. For example, when a client comes in saying "I'm depressed," elucidate specifics with questions such as:

- What do you mean when you say you are depressed?
- How do you recognize when you are depressed compared to when you are not?
- What changes indicate to you that you are depressed?

(Doran, 2013)

A mental health assessment contains two parts (Sadock & Sadock, 2010):

1. *Psychiatric History*: A record of the client's psychiatric history, so that the APMHN can understand the client better. Taking a thorough history enables the APMHN to make an accurate diagnosis and formulate an effective treatment plan.
2. *Mental Status Examination*: A description of the client's appearance, speech, actions, and thoughts, using a systematic format for recording findings about the client's thinking, feeling, and behavior. A client's history remains fixed, whereas their mental status can change during the interview, and these changes can be observable.

For example, during the engagement phase, the APMHN also starts to collect the following data for the same client's mental status:

- Appearance: Appeared to be the stated age, neatly groomed, wearing T-shirt and jeans, good hygiene.
- Speech: Soft spoken, logical, and rational.
- Mood: Sad and depressed.
- Affect: Tearful and mood congruent.

One of the common problems facing the novice APMHN is to determine which information in a full intake assessment is important, and how to prioritize urgent matters depending on the setting: emergency room for crisis intervention, hospital triage setting to determine the level of treatment, or outpatient setting for evaluation and treatment. In the emergency room or triage settings, the APMHN will only meet with the client once for a limited period of time, and therefore needs to conduct a highly structured interview with the goal of drawing a diagnostic impression and creating initial treatment plans. However, if the APMHN intends to see the client numerous times in an outpatient setting, then less data needs to be collected in the first interview, since further sessions are available before a treatment plan is created. Therefore, the APMHN's approach can be less structured and more relaxed, while collecting valid data to determine clinical impressions or possible diagnosis.

Phase 3: Closing of the Interview

Upon gathering sufficient data within the given time frame to determine the initial diagnosis and treatment plan, the APMHN will end the session by closing the interview, which consists of the actual closing words and gestures of the APMHN and of the client. Regardless of whether or not the APMHN will be seeing the client again, the APMHN should continue to be mindful of being warm and genuine rather than formal. The APHMN should also pay increased attention to the actions of the client at closing, as these may produce valuable information, especially if the APMHN will be seeing the client again. Shea (1998) claims that the closing of the interview may function as a mini-loss to the client. The client may respond with betrayal behaviors to such loss phenomenon, suggesting dependent feelings and difficulties with separation. These behaviors may be early signs of more far-reaching psychodynamic processes.

The final scenario presents the closing of the interview between the same client and the APMHN, and is followed by an analysis.

Client: I am glad that I came to see you today. I did not know what to expect, but I feel better after talking to you. Thank you.
APMHN: I am also glad that you sought help by coming to see me and that I was able to help. By the way, what was it about talking to me that helped you?

Comments: The client expressed appreciation (may view as dependence) as well as uncertainty. Since the betrayal by the boyfriend was the core issue, the APMHN should be keenly aware of psychodynamic processes, such as transference and countertransference, and maintain professional boundaries with the client.

Client: I don't know, just the way you allowed me to be myself, you did not judge me, and also, you were very patient with me. I felt like you understood my pain. … I did not even realize at the time that I was pouring my guts out. It's very unusual for me to do that to someone I've met for the first time.
APMHN: I am glad that I was helpful to you. It seems that you are ready to accept help and I am glad that you came today. Since we already talked about your

diagnosis and treatment plan, do you have any questions? And is it OK if we meet weekly for a while?

Comments: In the context of an initial mental health assessment of the client, the APMHN is required to create a record of the client's psychiatric evaluation, with a major goal being to identify signs and symptoms of psychiatric disorders, including other medical conditions that could affect the accuracy of a psychiatric diagnosis, as well as risk factors, such as suicidal, homicidal, or aggressive behaviors. Additional goals relate to identifying factors that could positively influence the therapeutic alliance, enhance clinical decision-making, enable safe and appropriate treatment planning, and promote better treatment outcomes. Finally, the initial psychiatric evaluation is the start of a dialogue between the APMHN and the client about many concerns, such as diagnosis and treatment options, and collaborative decision-making, including treatment-related decisions, as well as coordination of psychiatric treatment with other clinicians who may be involved in the client's care. These goals, which were delineated earlier, are all met by the end of the interview (Shea, 1998):

- Establish a sound engagement of the client in a therapeutic alliance.
- Collect a valid database.
- Develop an evolving and compassionate understanding of the client.
- Effect some decrease of anxiety in the client.
- Instill hope and ensure that the client will return for the next appointment.
- Develop an assessment from which a tentative diagnosis can be made.
- Develop an appropriate disposition and treatment plan.

Section 2: Guidelines of Mental Health Evaluation

In general, mental health assessment involves a structured interview with the client which depends on many factors, such as the client's ability to communicate, degree of cooperation, illness severity, and ability to recall historical details. Additional factors, such as past trauma (physical or sexual assault), different cultural backgrounds, primary language used, and mental health literacy, can influence the client's ability to establish trust within the therapeutic relationship. The APMHN's flexibility also may be needed to frame questions in a clearer manner. For example, during a mental health evaluation of a client with severe psychosis or dementia, obtaining information on psychiatric symptoms and history may not be possible through a structured interview with direct questioning (American Psychiatric Association [APA], 2016). In other words, during the mental health assessment, the APMHN should not be focused on following a rigid interview format but rather on formulating an appropriate structure that may even need to be adjusted as the assessment proceeds to guide the client and promote an effective therapeutic interview, while obtaining whatever needed clinical data is possible to obtain within a given time frame.

The APA (2016) delineates Practice Guidelines for the Psychiatric Evaluation of Adults as follows:

1. *History of Present Illness*
   - Reason that the patient is presenting for evaluation.
   - Psychiatric review of systems, including anxiety symptoms and panic attacks.
   - Past or current sleep abnormalities, including sleep apnea.
   - Impulsivity.
2. *Psychiatric History*
   - Past and current psychiatric diagnoses.
   - Prior psychotic or aggressive ideas, including thoughts of physical or sexual aggression or homicide.
   - Prior aggressive behaviors (e.g., homicide, domestic or workplace violence, other physically or sexually aggressive threats or acts).
   - Prior suicidal ideas, suicide plans, and suicide attempts, including aborted or interrupted ones, as well as details of each attempt (e.g., context, method, damage, potential lethality, intent).
   - Prior intentional self-injury in which there was no suicide intent.
   - History of psychiatric hospitalization and/or emergency department visits for psychiatric issues.
   - Past psychiatric treatments (type, duration, and, where applicable, doses).
   - Response to past psychiatric treatments.
   - Adherence to past and current pharmacological and nonpharmacological psychiatric treatments.
3. *Substance Use History*
   - Use of tobacco, alcohol, and other substances (e.g., marijuana, cocaine, heroin, hallucinogens) and any misuse of prescribed or over-the-counter medications or supplements.
   - Current or recent substance use disorders or change in use of alcohol or other substances.
4. *Medical History*
   - Allergies or drug sensitivities.
   - All medications the patient is currently or recently taking and any side effects (i.e., both prescribed and nonprescribed medications, herbal and nutritional supplements, and vitamins).
   - Whether or not the patient has an ongoing relationship with a primary healthcare professional.
   - Past or current medical illnesses and related hospitalizations.
   - Relevant past or current treatments, including surgeries, other procedures, or complementary and alternative medical treatments.
   - Past or current neurological or neurocognitive disorders or symptoms.
   - Physical trauma, including head injuries.
   - Sexual and reproductive history.
   - Cardiopulmonary status.

- Past or current endocrinological disease.
- Past or current infectious disease, including sexually transmitted diseases, HIV, tuberculosis, hepatitis C, and locally endemic infectious diseases, such as Lyme disease.
- Past or current symptoms or conditions associated with significant pain and discomfort.

5. *Review of Systems*
- Psychiatric (if not already included with history of present illness).
- Constitutional symptoms (e.g., fever, weight loss).
- Eyes.
- Ears, nose, mouth, throat.
- Cardiovascular.
- Respiratory.
- Gastrointestinal.
- Genitourinary.
- Musculoskeletal.
- Integumentary (skin and/or breast).
- Neurological.
- Endocrine.
- Hematological/lymphatic.
- Allergic/immunological.

6. *Family History*
- History of suicidal behaviors in biological relatives (for patients with current suicidal ideas).
- History of violent behaviors in biological relatives (for patients with current aggressive ideas).

7. *Personal and Social History*
- Presence of psychosocial stressors (e.g., financial, housing, legal, school/occupational, or interpersonal/relationship problems; lack of social support; painful, disfiguring, or terminal medical illness).
- Review of the patient's trauma history.
- Exposure to violence or aggressive behavior, including combat exposure or childhood abuse.
- Legal or disciplinary consequences of past aggressive behaviors.
- Cultural factors related to the patient's social environment.
- Personal/cultural beliefs and cultural explanations of psychiatric illness.
- Patient's need for an interpreter.

8. *Mental Status Examination*
- General appearance and nutritional status.
- Height, weight, and body mass index (BMI).
- Vital signs.
- Skin, including any stigmata of trauma, self-injury, or drug use.
- Coordination and gait.
- Involuntary movements or abnormalities of motor tone.
- Sight and hearing.

- Speech, including fluency and articulation.
- Mood, level of anxiety, thought content and process, and perception and cognition.
- Hopelessness.
- Current suicidal ideas, suicide plans, and suicide intent, including active or passive thoughts of suicide or death.
- If current suicidal ideas are present, assess:
  - Patient's intended course of action if current symptoms worsen.
  - Access to suicide methods, including firearms.
  - Patient's possible motivations for suicide (e.g., attention or reaction from others, revenge, shame, humiliation, delusional guilt, command hallucinations).
  - Reasons for living (e.g., sense of responsibility to children or others, religious beliefs).
  - Quality and strength of the therapeutic alliance.
- Current aggressive or psychotic ideas, including thoughts of physical or sexual aggression or homicide.
- If current aggressive ideas are present, assess:
  - Specific individuals or groups toward whom homicidal or aggressive ideas or behaviors have been directed in the past or at present.
  - Impulsivity, including anger management issues.
  - Access to firearms.

9. ***Impression and Plan***
   - Documentation of an estimate of the patient's suicide risk, including factors influencing risk.
   - Documentation of an estimated risk of aggressive behavior (including homicide), including factors influencing risk.
   - Quantitative measures of symptoms, level of functioning, and quality of life.
   - Documentation of the rationale for treatment selection, including discussion of the specific factors that influenced the treatment choice.
   - Asking the patient about treatment-related preferences.
   - An explanation to the patient of the following: the differential diagnosis, risks of untreated illness, treatment options, and benefits and risks of treatment.
   - Collaboration between the clinician and the patient about decisions pertinent to treatment.
   - Documentation of the rationale for clinical tests.

The APMHN formulates the basic structure of the interview by connecting each successive topic to the one that precedes it. For example, the earlier case scenario presented the topic of "breaking up with her boyfriend," which caused the client's emotional turmoil. Discussion of these issues led to the next phase of assessing the client's mental health status. The APMHN's ability to structure the interview naturally, transitioning organically from one phase to the next, requires a skillful approach, and the clinician's successful structuring lies in developing, understanding, and applying the contents of each heading of the mental health evaluation guidelines.

Section 3: Case Exemplar

Below is a sample psychiatric evaluation written by the APMHN at the conclusion of the case scenario presented earlier. The format used is slightly modified from the above APA (2016) guidelines to be practical for clinical use.

1. *Identification, Chief Complaint, and Reason for Referral*
    Jane Larson (JL) is a 31-year-old Caucasian female who presents with the chief complaint, "My family thinks I am depressed and need to see someone."
2. *History of Present Illness*
    JL reports that following the break-up 6 months ago with her boyfriend who was unfaithful to her, she has been isolating herself, crying a lot, not sleeping or eating, has poor concentration at work, is constantly preoccupied with the incident, and feels worthless and hopeless. JL also reports that she has been suffering from decreased motivation and low energy. She reports having thoughts recently of "just not being here," but denies having suicidal intent/plans. JL denies hallucinations, delusions, or homicidal ideations. JL wants to feel better so that she can move forward living her life.
3. *Past Psychiatric History*
    JL denies a history of psychotic symptoms and denies ever attempting to kill herself or having a history of psychiatric inpatient admission. Assessment revealed no history of manic episodes. JL reports intermittent treatment of depressive symptoms since her early 20s, typically provided by her primary care provider. She has been treated with either monotherapy antidepressants or a combination of antidepressants and benzodiazepine. Her treatment history also includes trials of sertraline, citalopram, venlafaxine XR, and bupropion. JL reports modest improvement of depressive symptoms with monotherapy of these antidepressants, which were, at times, supplemented with diazepam or lorazepam. JL has also received trazodone treatment for insomnia, which she reports as effective in the past. JL last received treatment for her mood symptoms 3 years ago. She states that she was not compliant with treatment for longer than 5 or 6 months because it did not seem to help her depression.
4. *Substance Use History*
    JL reports a history of using roughly one-half gram of marijuana two or three times weekly, "to take the edge off and help me to sleep." She does not drink alcohol or use other drugs.
5. *Social and Developmental History*
    JL is currently living alone, financially self-sufficient, and has a few close friends. She is the oldest of three siblings (two younger brothers) with whom she is not close. Father passed away when she was 5 years old and mother, who is 60 years old, has been supportive of her. JL denied any history of trauma.

6. ***Family Psychiatric History***

JL's family mental illness history is positive for depression (mother and maternal grandmother), and anxiety disorder (youngest brother). No one in JL's family has been admitted for inpatient psychiatric care. There is no family history of substance use disorder reported.

7. ***Medical History and Review of Systems***

JL's medical history is significant for hypothyroidism, seasonal allergies (pollen), and irritable bowel syndrome. Current medications include levothyroxine 0.75 mg daily. JL's surgical history includes a tonsillectomy at age 2, secondary to recurrent tonsillitis and ear infections. Review of systems showed no significant observable overall physical abnormalities. She is allergic to Demerol (nausea and vomiting).

8. ***Mental Status Examination***

   a. *General appearance*: Appeared to be the stated age, neatly groomed, wearing T-shirt and jeans, good hygiene. Soft spoken and cooperative during the interview.

   b. *Mood*: Sad and depressed.

   c. *Affect*: Tearful and mood congruent.

   d. *Thought content and process*: No significant thought disturbances noted. Denied current suicidal ideas, plans, and intent, including active or passive thoughts of suicide or death. Denied current aggressive or violent thoughts.

   e. *Perceptual disturbances*: Denied auditory, visual, or tactile hallucinations.

   f. *Sensorium, cognitive, and intellectual functioning*: Alert and oriented × 3. Attention span and concentration are intact, insight into the illness present.

9. ***Diagnostic Impression and Treatment Plan***

   a. *DSM-5 diagnosis*: Major depressive disorder (MDD), moderate. May use a patient health questionnaire (PHQ)-9 instrument to measure quantitative symptoms of depression.

   b. *Treatment plan*:
   - Assess current suicide risk, including ideation, intent, and plans.
   - Assess an estimated risk of aggressive behavior toward her ex-boyfriend.
   - Discuss treatment selections, including medication and psychotherapy, and ask the client about treatment-related preferences.
   - Explain to the client the following: differential diagnosis, risks of untreated illness, treatment options, and benefits and risks of treatment.

Section 4: Psychiatric Terminology

Review of Basic Psychiatric Terminology

Psychiatric terminology is commonly used to describe signs and symptoms of mental disorders. Signs of these disorders are usually objective observations of the client by the clinician, while symptoms are clients' subjective experiences. In the mental health field, signs and symptoms often overlap; therefore, mental disorders are described as syndromes—a constellation of signs and symptoms that together make up a recognizable condition (Sadock & Sadock, 2010). In the case scenario presented earlier, the client complains of symptoms of sadness, sleep disturbance, poor appetite, loneliness, and feeling down (depressed). The clinician observes signs of depressive disorder manifested by tearfulness, insomnia, weight loss, social isolation, and depressed mood. The clinician also observes and evaluates the client's mood, affect, speech, thought process and content, and sensory disturbance, and then documents the evaluation using appropriate terminology.

It is essential for APMHNs to be familiar with the basic psychiatric terminology commonly used to address these signs and symptoms so that they can fully implement and comprehend all psychiatric documentation utilized in clinical practice, including writing clients' psychiatric evaluations and communicating with other clinicians. The glossary of terms provided in Table 1.2 does not cover the full spectrum of psychiatric terminology, but is limited to commonly used basic terminology for APMHN students and clinicians to use as a quick reference.

Table 1.2 Glossary of Terms

Term	Definition
Aculalia	Nonsense speech associated with marked impairment of comprehension. Occurs in mania, schizophrenia, and neurological deficit (Sadock & Sadock, 2010).
Aerophagia	Excessive swallowing of air, usually an unconscious process associated with anxiety, resulting in abdominal distention or belching.
Affect	The subjective and immediate experience of emotion attached to ideas or mental representations of objects. Appropriate affect is emotional tone in harmony with the accompanying idea, thought, or speech. Affect that is not appropriate has outward manifestations that may be classified as:
	• Blunted affect: Severe reduction in the intensity of externalized feeling tone; one of the fundamental symptoms of schizophrenia.
	• Constricted affect: Reduction in intensity of feeling tone that is less severe than blunted affect.
	• Flat affect: Absence or near absence of any signs of affective expression.
	• Inappropriate affect: Emotional tone out of harmony with the idea, thought, or speech accompanying it. Seen in schizophrenia.
	• Labile affect: Affective expression characterized by rapid and abrupt changes, unrelated to external stimuli.
	• Restricted affect: Reduction in intensity of feeling tone that is less severe than in blunted affect but clearly reduced. May be used interchangeably with constricted affect.
Agnosia	Inability of a person to recognize faces, voices, places, or objects.
Agoraphobia	Morbid fear of open places or of leaving the familiar setting of the home. May be present with or without panic attacks.

(Continued)

Table 1.2 (Continued)

Term	Definition
Akathisia	Subjective feeling of motor restlessness manifested by a compelling need to be in constant movement; may be seen as an extrapyramidal adverse effect of antipsychotic medication. May be mistaken for psychotic agitation.
Alogia	Inability to speak due to mental deficiency or a manifestation of dementia.
Anergia	A chronic state of lethargy and low energy, commonly characterized by the inability to complete normal tasks. Often associated with depression.
Anhedonia	Loss of interest in, and withdrawal from, all regular and pleasurable activities. Inability to feel pleasure. A common symptom of depression as well as of other mental health disorders.
Anxiety	Feeling of apprehension caused by anticipation of danger, which may be internal or external. • Free-floating anxiety: Severe, pervasive, generalized anxiety that is not attached to any particular idea, object, or event. Observed particularly in anxiety disorders, although it may be seen in some cases of schizophrenia.
Apraxia	Inability to perform a voluntary purposeful motor activity despite being able to demonstrate normal muscle function. Apraxia is not related to a lack of understanding or to any kind of physical paralysis. Rather, it is caused by a problem in the cortex of the brain.
Blackout	Amnesia experienced by alcoholics about behavior during drinking bouts.
(Thought) Blocking	Abrupt interruption in train of thinking before a thought or idea is finished; after a brief pause, the person indicates no recall of what was being said or what was going to be said (also known as thought deprivation or increased thought latency). Common in schizophrenia and severe anxiety.
Catalepsy	Condition in which a person maintains the body position into which they are placed; observed in severe cases of catatonic schizophrenia. Also called *waxy flexibility*.
Circum-stantiality	Disturbance in associative thought and speech processes in which a person digresses into unnecessary details and inappropriate thoughts before communicating the central idea. Observed in schizophrenia, obsessional disturbances, and certain cases of dementia. See also **tangentiality**.
Clang association	Association or speech directed by the sound of a word rather than by its meaning; words have no logical connection; punning and rhyming may dominate the verbal behavior. Seen most frequently in schizophrenia or mania.
Concrete thinking	Thinking characterized by actual things, events, and immediate experience, rather than by abstractions.
Confabulation	Unconscious filling of gaps in memory by imagining experiences or events that have no basis in fact; commonly seen in amnestic syndromes. Should be differentiated from lying.
Coprolalia	Involuntary use of vulgar or obscene language. Observed in some cases of schizophrenia and in Tourette's syndrome.
Decompensation	Deterioration of psychic functioning caused by a breakdown of defense mechanisms. Seen in psychotic states.
Delirium	Acute reversible mental disorder characterized by confusion and some impairment of consciousness; generally associated with emotional lability, hallucinations or illusions, and inappropriate, impulsive, irrational, or violent behaviors.

(Continued)

Table 1.2 (Continued)

Term	Definition
Delusion	False belief, based on incorrect inference about external reality, that is firmly held despite objective and obvious contradictory proof or evidence, and despite the fact that other members of the culture do not share the belief. Types of delusions are:
	• Delusion of grandeur: Exaggerated conception of one's importance, power, or identity.
	• Delusion of persecution: False belief of being harassed or persecuted; often found in litigious patients who have a pathological tendency to take legal action because of imagined mistreatment. Most common delusion.
	• Delusion of reference: False belief that the behavior of others refers to oneself or that events, objects, or other people have a particular and unusual significance to the person, usually of a negative nature; derived from idea of reference, in which persons falsely feel that others are talking about them (e.g., belief that people on television or radio are talking to or about the person).
	• *Folie a deux*: Mental illness shared by two persons, usually involving a common delusional system; if it involves three persons, it is referred to as *folie a trois*, and so on.
	• Nihilistic delusion: Depressive delusion that the world and everything related to it has ceased to exist.
	• Somatic delusion: Delusion pertaining to the functioning of one's body.
	• Systemized delusion: Group of elaborate delusions related to a single event or theme.
Dysphoria	Feeling of unpleasantness or discomfort; a mood of general dissatisfaction and restlessness. Occurs in depression and anxiety.
Dystonia	Extrapyramidal motor disturbance consisting of slow, sustained contractions of the axial or appendicular musculature; one movement often predominates, leading to relatively sustained postural deviations; acute dystonic reactions (facial grimacing and torticollis) are occasionally seen with the initiation of antipsychotic drug treatment.
Echolalia	Psychopathological repeating of one person's words or phrases by another person; tends to be repetitive and persistent. Seen in certain kinds of schizophrenia, particularly the catatonic types.
Egocentric	Self-centered; selfishly preoccupied with one's own needs; little or no interest in others.
Euphoria	Exaggerated feeling of well-being that is inappropriate to real events. Can occur with drugs, such as opiates, amphetamines, and alcohol.
Formal thought disorder	Disturbance in the form, rather than in the content, of thought; thinking characterized by loosened associations, neologisms, and illogical constructs; thought process is disordered, and the person is defined as psychotic. Characteristics of schizophrenia. Types of formal thought disorders are:
	• Illogical constructs.
	• Loosened association.
	• Neologism.
Fugue	Dissociative disorder characterized by a period of almost complete amnesia, during which a person actually flees from an immediate life situation and begins a different life pattern; apart from the amnesia, mental faculties and skills are usually unimpaired.

(Continued)

Table 1.2 (Continued)

Term	Definition
Hallucination	False sensory perception occurring in the absence of any relevant external stimulation of the sensory modality involved. Types of hallucinations are • Auditory hallucination: False perception of sounds, usually voices, but also of other noises, such as music. Most common hallucination in psychiatric disorders. • Command hallucination: False perception of orders that a person may feel obliged to obey or unable to resist. • Gustatory hallucination: Hallucination primarily involving taste. • Olfactory hallucination: Hallucination primarily involving smell or odor; most common in medical disorders, especially in the temporal lobe. • Somatic hallucination: Hallucination involving the perception of a physical experience localized within the body. • Tactile hallucination (formication): Involving the sensation that tiny insects are crawling over the skin. Seen in cocaine addiction and delirium tremens. • Visual hallucination: Hallucination primarily involving the sense of sight.
Idea of reference	Misinterpretation of incidents and events in the outside world as having direct personal reference to oneself; occasionally observed in normal persons, but frequently seen in paranoid patients. If present with sufficient frequency or intensity, or if organized and systematized, they constitute delusions of reference.
Loosening of association	Unrelated and unconnected ideas, in which the person shifts from one subject to another. Characteristic schizophrenic thinking or speech disturbance involving a disorder in the logical progression of thoughts, manifested as a failure to adequately communicate verbally.
Mood	Pervasive and sustained feeling tone that is experienced internally and that, in the extreme, can markedly influence virtually all aspects of a person's behavior and perception of the world. Distinguished from affect, which is the external expression of the internal feeling tone. Types of mood, in order of severity: • Euthymia: Normal range of mood, implying absence of depression or of elevated mood. • Elevated mood: Air of confidence and enjoyment; a mood more cheerful than normal, but not necessarily pathological. • Exaltation: Feeling of intense elation and grandeur. • Expansive mood: Expression of feelings without restraint, frequently with an overestimation of their significance or importance. Seen in mania and grandiose delusional disorder. • Irritable mood: State in which one is easily annoyed and impatient, and provoked to anger. • Labile mood: Oscillations in mood between euphoria and depression or anxiety.
Neologism	New word or phrase whose derivation cannot be understood.
Paranoid ideation	Thinking dominated by suspicious, persecutory, or grandiose content of less than delusional proportions.
Preoccupation of thought	Centering of thought content on a particular idea, associated with a strong affective tone, such as a paranoid trend or a suicidal or homicidal preoccupation.

(Continued)

Table 1.2 (Continued)

Term	Definition
Psychomotor agitation	Physical and mental overactivity that is usually nonproductive and is associated with a feeling of inner turmoil, as seen in agitated depression.
Rumination	Constant preoccupation with thinking about a single idea or theme, as in obsessive-compulsive disorder (OCD).
Speech patterns	• Poverty of speech: Restriction in the amount of speech used; replies may be monosyllabic, little or no unprompted additional information provided. Occurs in major depression, schizophrenia, and organic mental disorders. Also called laconic speech. • Pressured speech: Increase in the amount of spontaneous speech; rapid, loud, accelerated speech. Occurs in mania, schizophrenia, and cognitive disorders. • Tangentiality: Oblique, digressive, or even irrelevant manner of speech in which the central idea is not communicated. • Word salad: Incoherent, essentially incomprehensible, mixture of words and phrases commonly seen in far-advanced cases of schizophrenia.
Suggestibility	State of uncritical compliance with influence, or of uncritical acceptance of an idea, belief, or attitude; commonly observed among persons with hysterical traits.
Suicidal ideation	Thoughts of taking one's own life.
Suicide attempt	A nonfatal, self-directed, potentially injurious behavior with any intent to die as a result of the behavior. A suicide attempt may or may not result in injury and may be aborted by the individual or interrupted by another individual.
Suicide intent	Subjective expectation and desire for a self-injurious act to end in death.
Thought disorder	Any disturbance of thinking that affects language, communication, or thought content; the hallmark feature of schizophrenia. Manifestations range from simple blocking and mild circumstantiality to profound loosening of association, incoherence, or delusions; characterized by a failure to follow semantic and syntactic rules that is inconsistent with the person's education, intelligence, or cultural background.

Source: Adapted from Sadock and Sadock (2010).

References

American Psychiatric Association (APA). (2016). *The American Psychiatric Association practice guidelines for the psychiatric evaluation of adults* (3rd ed.). American Psychiatric Association. https://doi.org/10.1176/appi.pn.2015.8a5

Belleza, M. (2020). Therapeutic communication techniques in nursing: Nurses-labs. https://nurseslabs.com/therapeutic-communication-techniques-in-nursing/

Doran, C. M. (2013). *Prescribing mental health medication: The practitioner's guide* (2nd ed.). Routledge. ISBN 9780415536097

Johnson, K., & Vanderhoef, D. (2016). *Psychiatric mental health nurse practitioner: Nursing certification review manual* (4th ed.). American Nurses Association. ISBN 978-193 521

Sadock, B., & Sadock, V. (2010). *Kaplan & Sadock's pocket handbook of clinical psychiatry* (5th ed.). Lippincott Williams & Wilkins.

Shea, S. C. (1998). *Psychiatric interviewing: The art of understanding* (2nd ed.). W.B. Saunders. ISBN-13: 978-0721670119

Walker, S. (2014). *Engagement and therapeutic communication in mental health nursing*. SAGE Publications. ISBN: 978 1 4462 7480 4

2 Case-Based Differential Diagnostic Mental Health Evaluation for Adults

Utilizing a common language with which to classify different psychiatric diagnoses enables mental health clinicians to facilitate a more consistent treatment and referral across practitioners. The two most recognized compilations of psychiatric classifications are the *Diagnostic and Statistical Manual of Mental Disorders* (DSM-5), published by the American Psychiatric Association (APA), and the International Classification of Diseases (ICD), developed by the World Health Organization (WHO). The DSM-5 (APA, 2013) is used in this book, as it is designed to facilitate reliable diagnoses by classifying mental disorders with associated criteria, and is therefore a standard reference for clinical practice in the mental health field.

The DSM-5 discusses 22 categories of psychiatric disorders; this chapter presents the ten most likely to be encountered by advanced psychiatric mental health nurses (APMHNs) in their clinical practice. For each, a case-based differential diagnostic mental health evaluation for adults is provided to demonstrate the common skills needed to achieve a successful evaluation and treatment plan. However, as this book is focused on assessment and diagnosis, each treatment plan is only presented briefly, tailored to the uniqueness of each disorder.

Furthermore, the language used in these case exemplars is not meant to be prescriptive. While there are essential aspects of an evaluation that must be covered to reach an accurate diagnosis, and while the APMHN should interact with clients in ways that allow them to feel comfortable enough to disclose essential information, each APMHN should adjust the language and style in these examples to fit their own personality, as that too is part of successful clinical practice.

Section 1: Schizophrenia

Schizophrenia is a psychotic disorder defined by the DSM-5 as the breakdown of an individual's perceptual, cognitive, and functional status to the point that the individual experiences reality in ways that are very different from how other people within the same culture experience it. It is the most common and best-known psychotic illness, but is not synonymous with psychosis. It affects 1% of the US population, with over 300,000 acute schizophrenic episodes in the United States annually (Stahl, 2013). Approximately 20% of clients diagnosed

DOI: 10.4324/9781003137597-3

with schizophrenia attempt suicide, and 5–6% of these eventually succeed (APA, 2013), contributing to a mortality rate that is eight times greater than that of the general US population. Life expectancy of a client with schizophrenia may be 20–30 years shorter than that of the general population due to multiple factors, such as poor physical health caused by smoking, unhealthy diet, obesity, or diabetes, some of which can be exacerbated by adverse reactions to antipsychotic medications (Stahl, 2013).

The syndrome of schizophrenia consists of a mixture of three major symptom categories—positive, negative, and cognitive—as presented in Table 2.1.

A diagnosis of schizophrenia involves a constellation of signs and symptoms associated with a client's occupational and social impairments.

Diagnostic Criteria

DSM-5 Schizophrenia Diagnostic Criteria Modified

A. **Signs and Symptoms:** Presents two (or more) of the following signs and symptoms, at least one of which must be 1, 2, or 3 below. Only one Criterion A symptom is required if delusions are bizarre or if hallucinations consist of either a voice keeping up or making a running commentary on the person's behavior or thoughts, or of two or more voices conversing with each other:
   1. Delusions.
   2. Hallucinations.
   3. Disorganized speech (e.g., frequent derailment or incoherence).
   4. Grossly disorganized or catatonic behavior.
   5. Negative symptoms (e.g., affective flattening, alogia, or anhedonia).
B. **Duration:** Each sign or symptom presents for a significant portion of time during a 1-month period (or less if successfully treated). Unless successfully treated, continuous signs of the illness persist for at least 6 months.

Table 2.1 Symptom Categories of Schizophrenia

Positive Symptoms	Negative Symptoms	Cognitive Symptoms
Delusions	Blunted affect	Problems representing and maintaining goals
Hallucinations	Emotional and apathetic social withdrawal	Problems focusing and sustaining attention
Distortions or exaggerations in language and communication	Passivity and poor rapport	Problems modulating behavior based upon social cues
Disorganized speech	Difficulty in abstract thinking	Problems prioritizing
Disorganized behavior	Lack of spontaneity	Problems with serial learning
Catatonic behavior	Alogia (restrictions in fluency and productivity of thought and speech)	Difficulty with problem-solving
Agitation	Anhedonia (lack of pleasure)	Impaired verbal fluency

Source: Adapted from Stahl (2013).

C. **Impairment in Function:** For a significant portion of the time following the onset of the illness, one or more major areas, such as work, interpersonal relations, or self-care, are markedly below the level achieved prior to the onset.

D. **Differential Diagnosis:** Rule out schizoaffective disorder and depressive or bipolar disorder with psychotic features by determining that:

1. No major depressive or manic episodes have occurred concurrently with the active phase symptoms.
2. If they have, they have been present for a minority of the total duration of the active and residual periods of the illness.

E. **Diagnostic Recording:** After 1-year duration of the disorder, the following specifiers can be used, as appropriate:

1. First episode, currently in acute episode.
2. First episode, currently in partial remission.
3. First episode, currently in full remission.
4. Multiple episodes, currently in acute episode.
5. Multiple episodes, currently in partial remission.
6. Multiple episodes, currently in full remission.
7. Continuous.
8. Unspecified.

In addition to understanding the DSM-5 diagnostic criteria for schizophrenia, it is essential that APMHNs have a working knowledge of its neurobiological basis, especially the role of brain circuits and related symptom dimensions, to accurately and safely prescribe psychotropic medications. Box 2.1 summarizes the neurobiological theories of schizophrenia from the currently available literature.

Box 2.1 Neurobiological Theories of Schizophrenia

While our understanding of the neurological basis of schizophrenia has advanced, leading to the development of more efficacious psychotropic medications, it is important to note that there are still many limitations to what is currently known, as every brain area has several functions, and every function is distributed across more than one brain area. However, ascribing specific symptom dimensions to unique brain areas not only assists research studies, but also has clinical value, as each client has unique psychiatric symptoms as well as specific responses to medications designed to target the brain's unique circuits, neurotransmitters, receptors, and enzymes.

A. Hypothesis of Neuroanatomy of Dopamine Neuronal Pathways in the Brain

The various symptoms of schizophrenia are hypothesized to be localized in the malfunctioning of unique brain regions. The neuroanatomy of dopamine (DA) neuronal pathways in the brain explains the symptoms of schizophrenia, as well as the therapeutic and adverse effects of antipsychotic medications. There are five dopamine pathways in the brain, two of which are predominantly related to positive and negative symptoms of schizophrenia: (1) the mesolimbic pathway's hyper-dopaminergic state, which results in positive symptoms; and (2) the mesocortical pathway's hypodopaminergic state, which results in negative, cognitive, and affective symptoms.

The **mesolimbic dopamine pathway** is involved in the regulation of emotional behaviors and is believed to be the predominant pathway that regulates positive symptoms of psychosis. Excessive dopamine activities in this pathway are believed to account for delusions and hallucinations. This pathway is also involved in pleasure, reward, and reinforcing behavior, and many drugs that are abused interact here.

The **mesocortical dopamine pathway** projects from the ventral tegmental area (VTA), followed by two separate projections in the prefrontal cortex (PFC): the dorsolateral prefrontal cortex (DLPFC) and the ventral medial prefrontal cortex (VMPFC). Projections specific to the DLPFC are associated with hypoactivity of dopamine neurons and are believed to be involved in the negative and cognitive symptoms of schizophrenia. Projections specific to the VMPFC are also associated with hypoactivity of dopamine neurons, but are believed to mediate negative and affective symptoms of schizophrenia.

Another key dopamine pathway in the brain is the **nigrostriatal dopamine pathway**, which projects from the brainstem substantia nigra through axons terminating in the basal ganglia or striatum. It is part of the extrapyramidal nervous system and plays a key role in regulating movements. It is believed that clients with schizophrenia do not have an abnormality of dopamine in this pathway. However, such a client taking antipsychotic medication which blocks dopamine may develop dopamine deficiency in this pathway, which can lead to extrapyramidal symptoms (EPS). In fact, chronic blockade of dopamine receptors in this pathway may result in a neuroleptic-induced tardive dyskinesia.

Another well-known dopamine pathway is the **tuberoinfundibular dopamine pathway**, in which dopamine neurons project from the hypothalamus to the anterior pituitary, where prolactin secretion into the blood circulation is regulated. Dopamine activity in this pathway is relatively preserved in clients with schizophrenia. However, as dopamine inhibits prolactin secretion, prolactin levels can rise, which leads to hyperprolactinemia in a client with schizophrenia who is treated with dopamine-blocking antipsychotic medication (Stahl, 2013).

There are currently two types of Food and Drug Administration (FDA)-approved pharmacologic options for the treatment of schizophrenia: (1)

dopamine blockers at dopamine receptors, to target the positive symptoms that typical antipsychotic medications (first-generation antipsychotics) target; and (2) antagonism at the serotonin (S-hydroxytryptamine, 5HT) receptor site to disinhibit dopamine release from the presynaptic dopamine neuron, which targets the negative, cognitive, and affective symptoms that atypical antipsychotic medications (second-generation antipsychotics) target. In other words, atypical antipsychotic medications are designed to block postsynaptic dopamine receptors in the mesolimbic pathway where dopamine antagonism is predominant, as well as to simultaneously promote the release of dopamine from the presynaptic dopamine neuron in the meso-cortical pathway, where less dopamine activity will take place (Citrome, 2011).

The dopamine neurotransmitter in the brain dopamine pathways related to symptoms of schizophrenia is summarized in Table 2.2.

Table 2.2 Dopamine Neurotransmitter Pathways and Level of Dopamine Resulting Symptoms of Schizophrenia

Brain Neurotransmitter Pathways	Level of Dopamine Neurotransmitter	Symptoms of Schizophrenia
Mesolimbic pathway; *from ventral tegmental area to nucleus accumbens*	Dopamine— hyper-dopa-minergic state	Positive symptoms
Mesocortical pathways; *from ventral tegmental area to cortex (dorsolateral prefrontal cortex [DLPFC] and the ventral medial prefrontal cortex [VMPFC])*	Dopamine— hypo-dopamin-ergic state	Cognitive symptoms (DLPFC) Negative symptoms (DLPFC and VMPFC) Affective symptoms (VMPFC)
Nigrostriatal pathway; *from the substantia nigra to the striatum*	Dopamine—sufficient	Dopamine blockade can lead to develop extrapyramidal symptoms (EPS)*
Tuberoinfundibular pathway; *from the hypothalamus to the pituitary gland*	Dopamine—sufficient	Dopamine blockade can lead to elevations in prolactin release*
Dopamine pathway arises from multiple sites; *from periaqueductal gray, ventral mesencephalon, hypothalamic nuclei, and lateral parabrachial nucleus to the thalamus*		Its function is not currently well known

Source: Stahl (2013).
Note: *Commonly known adverse reactions of antipsychotic medications are due to dopamine blockade.

B. Hypothesis of Glutamate Neurotransmitter Abnormality in the Brain

In addition to this well-known theory of dopamine neurotransmitter abnormalities in clients with schizophrenia, researchers have also explored the potential role of another brain neurotransmitter, glutamate, in the pathophysiology of schizophrenia, as a precursor to developing additional medications to treat it. **Glutamate is known as the major excitatory neurotransmitter** in the brain and is believed to interact with virtually all neurons in the brain that are involved in fast-synaptic transmission, in neuroplasticity, and in cognitive functions, including memory. In addition, glutamate neurons can be connected to dopamine neurons. Therefore, it is hypothesized that schizophrenia can be caused by hypofunctional glutamate activity at N-methyl-D-aspartate (NMDA) receptors due to abnormalities in the formation of glutamatergic NMDA synapses during neurodevelopment. This theory postulates that under normal circumstances, tonic inhibition occurs in the NMDA receptor regulation of the mesolimbic dopamine pathway (Stahl, 2013).

The glutamate neuron connects to a gamma aminobutyric acid (GABA) interneuron, which then connects to a dopamine neuron, resulting in the inhibition of dopamine release. In the presence of NMDA receptor hypofunction in the cortical brainstem projections of patients with schizophrenia, hyperactivity of the mesolimbic dopamine pathway would take place. In other words, in the normal state, glutamate acts as an indirect brake on dopamine release. However, hypoactive glutamate neurons result is insufficient

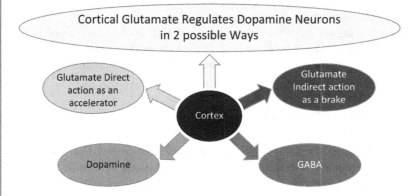

Figure 2.1 Cortical glutamate regulated dopamine neurons in two possible ways. Note: This figure shows the mechanism of how cortical glutamate regulates dopamine neurons in two possible ways; directly, by means of glutamatergic fibers projecting to the brainstem neurons (accelerator) and indirectly by fibers projecting to the glutamatergic/GABAergic pathway from cortex to brainstem (brake).

activity at the GABA interneuron, releasing the brake, which leads to excessive dopamine being released into the mesolimbic system, which produces the positive symptoms of schizophrenia. Cognitive, negative, and mood symptoms are explained by the possibility that glutamate neurons project directly on dopamine neurons, rather than through a GABA interneuron. Under normal conditions, NMDA receptor regulation of mesocortical dopamine pathways is that of tonic excitation, resulting in the release of sufficient dopamine in the DLPFC and VMPFC to allow successful regulation of cognition and mood, as well as avoiding so-called negative symptoms. With NMDA receptor hypofunction, the direct result would be hypoactivity of mesocortical dopamine pathways, with insufficient dopamine release in the DLPFC and VMPFC, resulting in the cognitive, negative, and affective symptoms of schizophrenia (Citrome, 2011) (Figure 2.1).

Interviewing Techniques to Assess Psychotic States of Schizophrenia

This section discusses practical points to help the APMHN assess a schizophrenic client's psychotic states and build a rapport with the client through understanding those states from the client's point of view. For example, assessing clients who experience auditory hallucinations can be challenging. APMHNs typically ask patients with known or suspected auditory hallucinations the following two questions: (a) "Do you hear voices?" and (b) "Are your voices commanding you to harm yourself or anyone else?" Although asking these questions is critically important to maintain the safety of these clients and others, additional questions should also be asked to obtain a comprehensive assessment of the clients' experiences with hallucinations (Trygstad et al., 2015).

The following are guidelines to assist the APMHN to effectively assess schizophrenic clients who exhibit one or both of the two most common major positive symptoms of schizophrenia: hallucinations (perceptual disturbances) and delusions (thought disturbances).

A. **Assessment of Hallucinations**

Shea (1998a) suggests that the following questions can convey to clients that the clinician is genuine in wanting to know about their experiences, while helping the clinician to learn about the contents of clients' hallucinations.

1. *When you are feeling very distressed, do your thoughts ever get so intense that they sound almost like a voice?*

    This question allows the clinician to tie the phenomena directly to the client's emotional turmoil in a fairly nonconfrontational fashion. Phrasing the client's thoughts as sounding like a voice can offer a back door to reluctant clients who fear being viewed as "crazy." If the client answers this question affirmatively, consider the following questions to gather further information.

2. *Tell me what the voices sound like to you.*
3. *What do they say to you?*
4. *Do they sometimes taunt you or say mean things about you?*
5. *Are they male or female voices?*
6. *Do they seem to be inside your head or do they come from outside your head?*

In a typical first interview, the APMHN may not have time to ask any or all of these questions, but as time permits in subsequent sessions, the clinician can pick and choose, constantly exploring to better understand the client's world and to assess their mental status while building a rapport with the client.

Additional questions can be asked to address potential risk factors and to find out if there are also nonauditory hallucinations.

1. *Do they ever tell you to harm yourself or others? (Important: risk, command hallucinations)*
2. *Have you had any strange tastes, smells, or visions lately? (Hallucinations in other modalities)*

B. Assessment of Thoughts and Delusions

1. *Have you ever felt/do you feel like your thoughts are being interfered with ... (pause) ... like thoughts are being put into your head? (Thought insertion)*
2. *Have you ever felt/do you feel like thoughts are being taken out of your head? (Thought withdrawal)*
3. *Have you ever felt/do you feel like your thoughts are being broadcast to other people so that they know what you are thinking? (Thought broadcasting)*
4. *Have you ever felt under the control of someone other than yourself?*
5. *Have you ever felt like your actions, feelings, or urges are being controlled by some external force? (Passivity phenomenon)*
6. *Have you ever felt any strange sensations in your body? (Somatic passivity)*
7. *Have you ever felt that people on the radio or TV were talking about you in their reports or giving you special messages? (Ideas or delusions of reference)*
8. *Do you ever receive any messages from books, radio, or TV that are specifically meant for you? (Paranoid bizarre delusions)*
9. *Do you ever feel like you are being spied upon or that someone is following you or conspiring against you? (Persecutory delusions)*
10. *Do you ever feel like you are being watched by cameras or special devices? (Persecutory delusions)*

Table 2.3 "Do" and "Do Not" Question Examples in Dealing with a Client with Delusions

Do Not	Dismiss their delusion as inconsequential
Do	**Calmly ask objective questions about their delusion**
Do Not	Verbally assault them or call them "crazy"
Do	**Seek medical attention for the individual should the situation warrant it**
Do Not	Play along with their delusion
Do	**Calmly ask in a nonjudgmental manner**

If the client answers "yes" to any of the above questions, the clinician can follow up with the question. *How did it start?* (to establish delusional perception).

(Retrieved from Psych Scene Hub (n.d.) Schizophrenia—Diagnostic Interview)

What is the best way to respond to someone experiencing delusions? Challenging these clients almost always causes them to put up their defenses and retreat further into their beliefs; however, feeding into their delusions will only give them more reason to think their beliefs are justified. Therefore, do not ignore the delusion or write it off as just a fleeting belief, but instead calmly ask the individual pertinent questions, such as the ones listed above, in a nonjudgmental manner to better understand their experiences and world. Furthermore, no matter how bizarre their answers may seem, simply listen without reacting one way or the other.

Table 2.3 provides examples of "Do" and "Do Not" ways in which the clinician should respond to the client's answers to their questions.

The following is a case exemplar of an initial psychiatric evaluation that demonstrates how the diagnosis of schizophrenia is determined, including the rationales and treatment plan for it.

Case Exemplar

The client's initials are KB.

A. *Identification, Chief Complaint, and Reason for Referral*

KB is a 51-year-old, English-speaking, Hispanic, divorced female who was brought to the emergency room (ER) by her son for a psychiatric evaluation and possible admission to the inpatient psychiatric unit. Her chief complaint is, "My son is conspiring against me and trying to lock me up in the hospital." As per her son, his mother needs to be admitted to the hospital because she decompensated due to medication noncompliance and it was becoming increasingly difficult to manage her at home.

B. *History of the Present Illness*

During the interview, KB stated, "I am doing well and feeling fine." The client verbalized paranoid and delusional ideations of being followed by unknown people and stated that her children are trying to poison her with medications. According to the client, she did not need to be admitted to the hospital and insisted that there were "powerful people" in the hospital who would hurt her. She expressed that she had to take action by "whistle blowing," because hospital staff were helping these "powerful people" and turning her children against her and making them admit her to the hospital. She also claimed that she had to stop taking medications because her family gave her "poisonous medications."

As per the patient's son, KB has been decompensating over the past 2 months since she stopped taking the medications; she was getting increasingly paranoid and delusional, and would not drink water if her son touched the glass. At times, she would barricade herself in her room at night, and has not been able to sleep for the last several nights. This morning, she called the police and reported that her son was injecting her with medications under her toenails. A police officer went to her apartment and suggested that her son bring her to the local ER. In the ER, she was agitated and yelling at the son, "Why do you listen to them? Why do you want to hurt me?" The client denied suicidal/homicidal ideations, and denies auditory, visual, or tactile hallucinations. The client's potential risk assessments were done with a general violence assessment and the Columbia-Suicide Severity Rating Scale; the results indicated low risk.

C. *Past Psychiatric History*

KB refused to provide her past psychiatric history and said, "They know everything about me here." According to the son, the patient has a long history of mental illness and has been hospitalized multiple times in different hospitals in New York City. The son stated that his mother's first episode of the illness was in her late 20s and since then she has been hospitalized intermittently. She has been prescribed different neuroleptics, but as per the son's report, the best results were from Zyprexa (Olanzapine), which she stopped taking approximately 2 months ago. The medical records of previous admissions to the hospital were retrieved and reviewed. Findings indicated multiple admissions to the inpatient psychiatric unit: on 6/16/2008, 3/4/2009, 7/28/2013, 2/18/2015, 9/01/2017, and 10/15/2018. During each admission, the patient presented with paranoid delusions, basically due to noncompliance with medications. During the last admission, she presented with symptoms of paranoid delusions similar to this time, accusing her brothers, sisters, and sons of having malicious intention to hurt her and lock her up. She was admitted to the inpatient psychiatric unit on an involuntary status. She stabilized once the medications were resumed and was discharged ten days later.

D. *Substance Use History*

KB denied any history of substance use and the family confirmed the same. A urine toxicology was done, and the result was negative.

E. *Social and Developmental History (supplemental information was obtained from the client's previous medical records)*

KB is residing with her two sons, who are supportive and understanding of her chronic mental illness. But she has alienated herself from other relatives and friends. KB denied any history of trauma, such as exposure to violence or childhood abuse.

1. *Education*: KB dropped out of high school in eleventh grade, and later obtained her General Education Diploma (GED) certificate.
2. *Family Relationship, Social Network, and Abuse History*: KB was born in Puerto Rico and moved to New York City when she was 1 week old. She is the youngest of five siblings and several step-siblings, with whom she is not close. Her mother died when she was young; her father left the family soon after her birth. She was raised by her uncle, who sexually and physically abused her. She was married for 11 years to a physically abusive man and has two sons. She is divorced and resides with her sons in an apartment building in Brooklyn.
3. *Employment Record*: KB has had various jobs: cashier at different supermarkets, salesperson at a bridal shop, helper at a laundromat. However, due to her mental illness, she has not been able to work since 2000 and is currently on disability.
4. *Legal Records*: KB denies any problem with the law and denies any criminal records.
5. *Religious Background*: KB considers herself to be Catholic, but has not been an active member of any Catholic church and has not participated regularly in religious services.

F. **Family Psychiatric History**

As per KB's report, her mother is deceased of unknown etiology, the father has a history of alcohol abuse, and her sister has been on medications for chronic psychosis. KB was not able to provide any additional details of family mental illness history. She denied any family history of suicidal or violent behaviors.

G. **Medical History and Review of Systems**

1. No known allergies (NKA) or drug sensitivities.
2. No significant past or current medical illnesses reported, and has not seen her primary care provider (PCP) for a regular physical examination in over a year.
3. Overall, no significant observable physical abnormalities are noted via a review of systems, except for the son's report that she is not eating regularly due to her paranoia and has lost 3–4 lbs within the last month or so.
4. Vital signs: BP: 108/68; HR: 77; RR: 18; Temp: 36.6 C; Ht: 5'5"; Wt: 110 lbs; body mass index [BMI]: 18.3.

H. **Mental Status Examination**

1. *Appearance and Behavior*: KB appears to be the stated age; general appearance is disheveled with poor hygiene; overall behavior is partially

cooperative with poor eye contact during the interview; her speech demonstrates fluency in English and Spanish, with a rapid and pressured
speech pattern, and tangential and circumstantial thoughts.

2. *Mood*: Labile, varying from angry and tearful to laughing.
3. *Affect*: Irritable, guarded, and suspicious.
4. *Thought Content and Process*: Presence of paranoia and delusions with
   flight of ideas. Denied current suicidal ideas, plans, and intent, including
   active or passive thoughts of suicide or death. Denied current aggressive
   or violent thoughts.
5. *Perceptional Disturbances*: Denied auditory, visual, and tactile
   hallucinations.
6. *Sensorium, Cognitive, and Intellectual Functioning*: KB is alert and oriented × 3. Attention span and concentration are limited, no insight into
   the illness with poor judgment. However, intellectual functioning is on
   average level.

I. **Diagnosis and Treatment Plan**

1. **DSM-5 Diagnosis**: Schizophrenia, multiple episodes, currently in acute
   episode.
2. **Rationale for Diagnostic Impression**: According to the DSM-5 (APA,
   2013), the following criteria must be present to diagnose schizophrenia.
   KB meets those criteria, as indicated by the bold symptom categories:

A. *Two (or more) of the following symptoms, each present for a significant
   portion of time during a 1-month period (or less if successfully treated). At
   least one of these must be 1, 2, or 3*:
   1. **Delusions.** KB manifested symptoms of paranoid delusions by not drink-
      ing water if her son had touched the glass, as she was afraid of being poi-
      soned; by barricading herself in her room at night; and by not being able to
      sleep for the last several nights due to the belief that her family would harm
      her. The morning of the evaluation, she called the police and reported that
      her son was injecting her with medications under her toenails.
   2. Hallucinations.
   3. **Disorganized speech** (e.g., frequent derailment or incoherence). KB's
      speech was incoherent and irrational, as evidenced by frequent jumping
      from one topic to another during the interview.
   4. Grossly disorganized or catatonic behavior.
   5. Negative symptoms (i.e., diminished emotional expression or avolition).
B. *For a significant portion of time since the onset of the disturbance, the
   level of functioning in one or more major areas, such as work, interpersonal relations, or self-care, is markedly below the level achieved prior to
   onset.* KB presented a long history of mental illness starting in her late 20s,
   with multiple hospitalizations secondary to medication noncompliance. Due
   to her mental health illness, she has not been able to work since 2000 and is
   currently on disability.

C. ***Continuous signs of the disturbance persist for at least 6 months. This 6-month period must include at least 1 month of symptoms (or less if successfully treated) that meet Criterion A.*** KB's symptoms returned each time she stopped her medications, leading to multiple hospitalizations, including this one; she stopped her medications 2 months ago and decompensated, with persecutory paranoid delusions and behavioral disturbances.

D. Schizoaffective disorder and depressive or bipolar disorder with psychotic features have been ruled out because either (1) no major depressive or manic episodes have occurred concurrent with the active-phase symptoms, or (2) if mood episodes have occurred during the active-phase symptoms, they have been present for a minority of the total duration of the active and residual periods of the illness.

E. The disturbance is not attributable to the physiological effects of substance use (e.g., a drug or medication) or another medical condition.

F. If there is a history of autism spectrum disorder or a communication disorder of childhood onset, the additional diagnosis of schizophrenia is made only if prominent delusions or hallucinations, in addition to the other required symptoms of schizophrenia, are present for at least 1 month (or less if successfully treated).

KB presented no history of major depressive or manic episodes and her symptoms did not appear to be attributable to the physiological effect of substance use or of medical conditions. She has no history of autism spectrum disorder or of a communication disorder of childhood onset.

Therefore, KB's diagnostic impression meets the criteria for schizophrenia with specifier—multiple episodes, currently in acute episode.

3. ***Treatment Plan***: Explain to the client and the family the appropriate treatment plan, including the diagnostic impression, risks of untreated illness, treatment options, benefits and risks of treatment, and the client treatment-related preferences:

- *Level of care*: Inpatient hospitalization. Currently, KB presents an acute episode of schizophrenia with paranoid delusions and the inability to care for self, and has no insight into her psychiatric conditions. Consequently, her level of functioning and quality of life have been compromised and, with the family's consent, hospitalization is recommended for her safety.

- *Risk assessment* of violence and aggressive behaviors toward self and/or others should be done to monitor potential harm.

- *Family involvement* in the treatment plan, including the option of long-acting antipsychotic medication to reduce medication noncompliance, and exploring potential community and social supports to alleviate the burden on the family and reduce KB's social isolation.

- *Medications*: Resume antipsychotic medications, as they are effective and were well-tolerated in the past. KB has a history of responding well to atypical antipsychotic medication (Zyprexa), which she tolerates well with no adverse reactions, but decompensated following medication noncompliance. Therefore, the same medication would be recommended. Zyprexa (Olanzapine) is a second-generation antipsychotic medication, designed to block postsynaptic dopamine receptors in the mesolimbic pathway, where dopamine antagonism is predominant, and to simultaneously promote the release of dopamine from the presynaptic dopamine neuron in the mesocortical pathway in the brain, where less dopamine activity takes place.

Section 2: Depressive Disorders

As shown in the previous section, the search for a diagnosis entails more than simply determining what it is; through the process of conducting a diagnostic interview, the APMHN aims to understand the manner in which the client experiences the world. Therefore, this section will emphasize the search for an understanding of depressive phenomena, exploring more fully the impact that symptoms inflict on the depressed individual's life, and that same process can and should be utilized for other mental health disorders as well. In terms of depression specifically, the more the APMHN understands that it is a process that constantly unfolds and manifests in phenomena that affect numerous systems outside the depressed individual, the more the clinician can sharpen their interviewing skills to catch the subtle clues suggesting depression. Ultimately, the APMHN's sensitivity will be enhanced, as will the therapeutic engagement with clients.

Depressive disorders as a primary diagnosis for adults are categorized in the DSM-5 (APA, 2013) as (1) major depressive disorder (MDD), including a major depressive episode, which is considered the classic condition in this group of disorders; (2) persistent depressive disorder (dysthymia); and (3) premenstrual dysphoric disorder. The common feature of all these disorders is the presence of sad, empty, or irritable mood, accompanied by somatic and cognitive changes that significantly affect the person's capacity to function. What differs among them are issues of duration, timing, or presumed etiology (Table 2.4).

MDD is one of the most prevalent mental disorders worldwide; lifetime prevalence rates range between 8% and 12% for most countries (Kessler & Bromet,

Table 2.4 Differential Diagnosis among Depressive Disorders in Adults Based on Duration

Diagnosis	Duration
Major depressive disorder	A minimum of 2 weeks
Persistent depressive disorder	A minimum of 2 years
Premenstrual dysphoric disorder	Begins following ovulation and remits within a few days of menses

2013). In the United States, the 12-month prevalence rate is approximately 7%, and the prevalence rate in 18- to 29-year-old individuals is three times that of those aged 60 years or older. Women experience 1.5–3.0 times higher rates than do men (APA, 2013). A National Center for Health Statistics (NCHS) survey reported that in 2019, 18.5% of adults had symptoms of depression, lasting at least 2 weeks, that were either mild, moderate, or severe (see E3 below), and that women were more likely than men to experience depressive symptoms. A study by Villarroel and Terlizzi (2020) indicated that the percentage of adults who experienced any symptoms of depression was highest among those aged 18–29 (21.0%), followed by 45–64 (18.4%), 65 and over (18.4%), and 30–44 (16.8%).

In this section, MDD, the most prevalent depressive disorder, will be used as an example to address mental status assessment and diagnostic evaluation for depressive disorders more broadly.

Diagnostic Criteria

DSM-5 (APA, 2013) Major Depressive Disorder
Diagnostic Criteria Modified

A. **Signs and Symptoms:** Presents five (or more) of the following signs and symptoms nearly every day, including at least Criterion 1 or 2:
   1. Depressed mood most of the day, subjective report of feeling sadness, emptiness, hopelessness, or observation made by others, such as tearful appearance.
   2. Markedly diminished interest or pleasure in all, or almost all, activities most of the day.
   3. Appetite-related significant weight change (more than 5% of body weight loss or gain in a month) when not dieting.
   4. Sleep disturbance (insomnia or hypersomnia).
   5. Psychomotor agitation or retardation.
   6. Fatigue or loss of energy.
   7. Feelings of worthlessness or excessive or inappropriate guilt.
   8. Diminished ability to think or concentrate, or indecisiveness.
   9. Recurrent thoughts of death, recurrent suicidal ideation without a specific plan, or a suicide attempt or a specific plan for committing suicide.
B. **Duration:** Five (or more) of the above signs or symptoms present during the same 2-week period, representing a change from previous functioning.
C. **Impairment in Function:** The symptoms cause clinically significant distress or impairment in social, occupational, or other important areas of functioning.
D. **Differential Diagnosis:** Careful consideration should be given to the delineation of normal sadness and grief from a major depressive episode. For example, bereavement may induce great suffering, but it does not typically induce an episode of MDD. In distinguishing grief from a major depressive episode, it is useful to consider that in grief, the predominant affect is feelings

of emptiness and loss, while in a major depressive episode it is persistent depressed mood and the inability to anticipate happiness or pleasure.

E. **Diagnostic Recording:** In recording the name of a diagnosis, terms should be listed in the following order for clinical consistency:
1. Major depressive disorder.
2. Single or recurrent episode.
3. Severity specifiers: Current severity specifiers are based on the number of criterion symptoms, the severity of those symptoms, and the degree of functional disability:
   a. *Mild*: Few symptoms in excess of those required to make the diagnosis are present, symptom intensity is distressing but manageable, and the symptoms result in minor impairment to social or occupational functioning.
   b. *Moderate*: The number of symptoms, intensity of symptoms, and/or functional impairment are between those specified for "mild" and "severe."
   c. *Severe*: The number of symptoms is substantially in excess of that required to make the diagnosis, symptom intensity is seriously distressing and unmanageable, and the symptoms markedly interfere with social and occupational functioning.

In addition to understanding the DSM-5 diagnostic criteria for depressive disorders, it is essential that APMHNs have a working knowledge of its neurobiological basis, especially the role of brain circuits and related symptom dimensions, to understand how psychotropic medications are used in its treatment. Box 2.2 summarizes the neurobiological theories of depressive disorders.

Box 2.2 Neurobiological Theories of Depressive Disorders

From a clinical perspective, the most influential neurobiological discoveries related to depression have probably been neurotransmitter-related abnormalities, with the monoamines (serotonin, noradrenaline, and dopamine) having received most attention in the development of antidepressants to relieve depressive symptoms. Yet, despite the current primary focus on monoamines, there is accumulating evidence that changes in other neurotransmitter systems can also be associated with depression, specifically the gamma aminobutyric acid (GABA) system (Kaltenboeck & Harmer, 2018).

Monoamine hypothesis

The classic theory about the neurobiological etiology of depression hypothesizes that it is due to a deficiency of three key monoamine neurotransmitters (serotonin, norepinephrine [NE], and dopamine), which may lead to malfunctioning of information processing in various brain regions. Currently, the monoamine hypothesis of depression is applied to understand how monoamine regulates the efficiency of information processing in a wide variety of neuronal circuits in the specific brain regions that may be responsible for medicating the various symptoms of depression (Stahl, 2013).

Table 2.5 presents each of the nine symptom criteria listed in the DSM-5 to diagnose an individual's MDD, hypothetically associated with the functionality of each brain region.

There are many brain areas where the key neurotransmitters' (serotonin, norepinephrine, and dopamine) projections overlap, creating opportunities for monoamine interactions throughout the brain (see Table 2.2). The monoamine hypothesis of depression posits that if a sufficient amount of monoamine neurotransmitter activity becomes reduced, depleted, or dysfunctional, depression may ensue. Numerous known inter-regulatory pathways and receptor interactions exist among the three monoaminergic neurotransmitter systems that enable them to influence each other and change the release not only of their own neurotransmitters, but also of other monoamines (Stahl, 2013). However, direct evidence of this hypothesis is still largely lacking. Regardless, a basic understanding of these neurotransmitters' projection pathways in the brain regions associated with symptoms of depression (as shown in Table 2.6) will build a strong foundation for the APMHN to translate neurobiological theories into clinical practice.

Table 2.5 Nine Symptom Criteria of Major Depressive Disorder and Associated Brain Regions Listed in the DSM-5

Symptom Criteria of Major Depression Disorder	Brain Regions
Depressed mood	Prefrontal cortex (PFC)
Diminished interest or pleasure	Nucleus accumbens (NA)
Appetite-related body weight loss or gain	Hypothalamus (HY)
Sleep disturbance (insomnia or hypersomnia)	Hypothalamus (HY)
	Basal forebrain (BF)
	Thalamus (T)
Psychomotor agitation or retardation	Prefrontal cortex (PFC)
	Cerebellum (C)
Fatigue or loss of energy	Striatum (S)
	Spinal cord (SC)
Feelings of worthlessness or excessive or inappropriate guilt	Prefrontal cortex (PFC)
	Amygdala (A)
Diminished ability to think or concentrate, or indecisiveness	Prefrontal cortex (PFC)
	Hippocampus (H)
Recurrent thoughts of death, recurrent suicidal ideation/plan/attempt	Prefrontal cortex (PFC)
	Amygdala (A)

Table 2.6 Three Key Neurotransmitters' Projection Pathways Associated with Symptoms of Depression

Neurotransmitter	Projection Origin	Projection Terminal	Symptoms of Depression
Serotonin (5HT)		PFC, BF, S,	Regulate mood, anxi-
• Ascending	Brain stem	NA, T,	ety, sleep, arousal,
		HY, A, H,	cognition, and other
		NT, C	functions listed in
			Table 2.1
• Descending	Brain stem	SC	Regulate pain pathways
Norepinephrine (NE)		PFC, BF, T,	Regulate mood, arousal,
• Ascending	Locus coeruleus of the brain stem	HY, A, H, NT, C	cognition, and other functions listed in Table 2.1
• Descending	Locus coeruleus of the brain stem	SC	Regulate pain pathways
Dopamine (DA)		Extend via H	See the dopamine-
• Widespread ascending projection	Brain stem partially ventral tegmental and substantia nigra	to PFC, BF, S, NA, and PFC, BF, T, HY, A, H	associated psychotic symptoms
• Other projections	Thalamus dopaminergic system	Thalamus	Arousal and sleep

Source: Adapted from Stahl (2013).

Neurotrophic hypothesis

The neurotrophic hypothesis of depression is based on the assumption that monoamine signaling and brain-derived neurotrophic factor (BDNF) release play a role in the proper growth and maintenance of neurons and neuronal connections (Stahl, 2013). Studies have highlighted a potential role for BDNF to contribute to the pathophysiology of depression, which may be caused by reduced synthesis of proteins involved in neurogenesis and synaptic plasticity. And treatment of depression is based on the assumption that antidepressant affect on BDNF expression in cortical and subcortical brain regions is implicated in reversing neuronal atrophy, neurogenic decline, and enhanced despair (Jaggar et al., 2019). A hyperactivation of the hypothalamic–pituitary–adrenal (HPA) axis has been found in 50% of depressed patients, and a significant decrease of BDNF levels has been demonstrated in depressed patients (Guerrera et al., 2020).

Glutamate hypothesis

Despite the availability of multiple classes of drugs that act upon monoamine-based mechanisms, studies indicate that at least 20–30% of subjects do not attain early improvement or remission after 4–12 weeks of treatment and fail to achieve a sustained remission of depressive symptoms (De Vries et al., 2019). The focus for improved pharmacotherapies for treatment-resistant depression, thus, has shifted to a neuroplasticity hypothesis focused on gluta-mate, which represents a substantial advancement in the working hypothesis that drives research for new drugs and therapies. In particular, studies show-ing that the glutamatergic modulator ketamine elicits fast-acting, robust, and relatively sustained antidepressant, antisuicidal, and antianhedonic effects in individuals with treatment-resistant depression have prompted interest in understanding the mechanisms responsible for ketamine's clinical effi-cacy (Kadriu et al., 2019). Much of this interest revolves around glutamate's role in regulating synaptic connectivity and signaling mechanisms by either inhibitory or excitatory proteins. It is based on the belief that during synaptic formation, a burst of glutamate is released, activating postsynaptic recep-tors, which in turn trigger downstream pathways that influence dendritic spine density, synaptic formation, and connectivity (Stahl, 2013).

Interviewing Techniques in Assessment of Depressive Disorders

As discussed in Shea's (1998) *Psychiatric Interviewing*, to fully understand depres-sion in the initial interview, depressed clients' experiences can be compartmental-ized into various subsystems: (1) physiologic system, (2) psychological system, (3) dyadic system, and (4) family and other group systems, each of which should be explored to the extent possible to enable the APMHN to make an accurate diagnosis.

1. Physiologic system is applied to the following DSM-5 signs and symp-toms of depression: appetite and sleep disturbances, psychomotor agitation or retardation, and fatigue or loss of energy. These experiences of altered functioning can become immensely disturbing to the client. With the client's experiences in mind, the following samples of clinician questions may add depth to the interview:
   a. What has your body felt like to you recently?
   b. What does it feel like to you to have lost your energy and drive?
   c. Do you feel that you have lost your energy, your appetite, and your abil-ity to sleep for the past 2 weeks?
   d. How have all these changes made you feel about yourself?

These types of questions not only allow a client the chance to vent, but also emphasize that the APMHN is interested in them as a unique individual whose depression they alone can explain.

2. Alteration in psychological system is divided into four broad areas, with each area linked to DSM-5 diagnostic symptoms and recommended clinician approaches. See Table 2.7 for a detailed explanation of each.

Table 2.7 Psychological Systems Linked to DSM-5 Diagnostic Symptoms and Recommended Clinician Approaches

Psychological Area	DSM-5 Diagnostic Symptom Criteria	Recommended Clinician Approach
Perception of the world	Depressed mood with feelings of sadness, emptiness, hopelessness	To fully grasp a feature of the depressed client's perception of their world, the clinician needs to enter the depressed client's world as best as possible; at times, when the client has difficulty in responding, the clinician needs to be more active while accepting the client's difficulty with patience
Cognitive processes	Diminished ability to think or concentrate, or indecisiveness, along with rumination and worries about the past, the present, and the future	Acknowledge the client's thoughts and allow them to vent while simultaneously refocusing the client's thinking process
Thought content	Thoughts of worthlessness or excessive or inappropriate guilt, along with loneliness, self-loathing, hopelessness, and helplessness Recurrent thoughts of death, recurrent suicidal ideation without a specific plan, or a suicide attempt or a specific plan for committing suicide	The clinician needs to be keenly aware of the potential risk of suicide; depending on the severity of these symptoms, probing with the following questions may help the clinician to assess the intensity of suicidal risk: "At this time, what kinds of ways of getting help do you see for yourself?" and "What do you see for yourself in the future?"; if needed, consider using a suicide assessment instrument, such as the Columbia-Suicide Severity Rating Scale (C-SSRS)
Psychodynamic defenses	This part is not included in the DSM-5 symptom criteria. But these defenses are common among depressed clients, such as denial, repression, rationalization, or isolation	Careful questioning will often uncover the depression by eliciting neurovegetative symptoms or evidence of depressive cognitive functioning

3. A dyadic system is created when two people interact. Depression, though, alters the interpersonal field; symptoms of depression, such as lack of motivation, social isolation, or avoidance, decrease the quality of a person's interaction with others, who in turn may treat the depressed person with reservation. Alternately, the dyadic system of the depressed person may be restricted, diminishing the chance to gain positive reinforcement from others and consequently creating a world lacking in reward for interactions with others. This unhealthy cycle of the dyadic system in the depressed person can lead to a learned helplessness, in which the depression ensures its own survival.

The APMHN can search for evidence of disturbances in the depressed client's dyadic system and of learned helplessness with the following questions:

a. Do you find yourself going out as frequently as you used to?
b. Tell me what it is like for you when you are around people at work?
c. When you talk with people, what kinds of feelings do you have, for instance if you meet a friend on the street?
d. How do people seem to be treating you?
e. Do you find yourself easily irritated or "flying off the handle" recently?
f. Does it require much energy to be around people, such as your friends?

It is important for the APMHN to be aware that not only are the client's family and friends affected by the client's depression, but the treating clinician may be as well. It is therefore beneficial for the APMHN to periodically reflect on their own emotional responses by:

a. Being keenly aware of their own negative and/or positive feelings, including overly empathic feelings toward a depressed client, which can seriously damage the therapeutic engagement, and/or
b. Adjusting to the needs of the client by utilizing continuous and adaptive creativity.

For example, when interviewing crying clients, the APMHN can be both empathic and professional, as demonstrated by the following responses:

#1 Client: (Tears coming down, but obviously trying not to cry.)
APMHN: "You seem sad right now. Are you trying not to cry?" (Said with a soft tone and also offering the client a chance to vent, thus decreasing a sense of discomfort.)
#2 Client: (Uncontrollable crying.)
APMHN: "What you are going through is obviously very upsetting and would be to anybody. Take a moment to collect yourself. It's important for us to talk more about what has happened to you."

In both situations, training in self-reflection by searching for answers to questions, such as the following, may enhance the APMHN's interviewing skills:

- What do I feel when someone cries?
- Do I ever perceive crying people as weak or ineffectual?
- How often do I cry and how do I feel about myself when I do?
- Have I ever seen my parents, family, or friends cry, and how did I feel then?

Generally acknowledged emotions commonly felt by clinicians are sympathy, empathy, and a desire to help. Additionally, a clinician's training in how to effectively recognize and deal with transference and countertransference will enhance their ability to effectively deal with the client's emotions.

4. Family and other group systems are important dynamics for the APMHN to explore to understand how the client's depression may affect other aspects of their life, such as the job environment or social organizations.

The impact of depression on family members and/or significant others, if any, is usually assessed in the initial interview. Family tensions may be spontaneously brought up by the client. At other times, skillful questions may be needed to illuminate these issues. Sample questions such as the following may be a good start:

a. Who in your family seems to understand you?
b. Who in your family are you concerned about right now?
c. How do you think your family members view your depression?
d. What kinds of suggestions have your family members been making to you about how to feel better?
e. What kinds of pressures has your spouse or partner been coping with recently?

Probing but open-ended questions, such as the above, will often yield information about the state of the family and may elicit interpersonal tensions toward specific family members, whereas more direct questions might elicit denial. Additionally, through this type of questioning, the APMHN may also learn valuable information about situational stressors in the family system.

Reflections of depression can be seen in group systems affected by changes in the client, such as a job environment or social networks (e.g., conflict with supervisor, poor performance at the job, avoidance of going out with friends). In addition, a disturbance in one system may affect other systems by acting as a major stressor which triggers the depression, as well as leaving its mark throughout all these interlocking systems (e.g., loss of a house from natural disaster leading to financial constraints).

The following is a sample case exemplar of the initial psychiatric evaluation, including how the diagnosis of MDD is determined, along with the proposed treatment plan and rationales.

Case Exemplar

The client's initials are JO.

A. *Identification, Chief Complaint, and Reason for Referral*

JO is a 35-year-old, Hispanic, single mother with a 17-year-old son and 5-year-old twin sons. She is currently employed as a medical assistant and has been working at the same clinic for the past 13 years. She was referred to the mental health clinic by the twin sons' therapist and presents with the chief complaint "I feel unorganized and drained." She is well groomed and neatly dressed in her uniform from work.

B. *History of Present Illness*

JO reported that she has been grieving the loss of her mother, who passed away a year ago. She has also been under a lot of stress due to losing a potential new career opportunity to be a police officer, an ongoing battle with the father of her twin sons, who left 2 years ago, and dealing with her twin sons' behavioral problems due to attention deficit hyperactivity disorder (ADHD).

JO stated that since the death of her mother, she has been disorganized and feeling totally drained physically. She grieves every day, misses her all the time, has difficulty accepting the mother's death, and still exhibits disbelief that she is gone. JO claimed that she has been crying all the time and avoiding visiting the mother's apartment, where her brother now resides. She reports loneliness and has detached herself from her siblings, stating, "my circle of surroundings just gets smaller and smaller." She also expressed great disappointment over being rejected by the police academy, where she had studied and trained for a long time to become a police officer, due to an incident of smoking marijuana once last summer. She admitted to having a substance use problem, but maintained that she had been abstinent for 5 years until this one episode. An additional stress is that both of her twin sons were diagnosed with ADHD and have behavioral problems at school; the teacher has reported that they kick and hit other children, and also cry and hit themselves. JO stated that dealing with all these issues has left her feeling exhausted and with no energy, and reported eating more and gaining weight (7 lbs within 2 months). She no longer does things she used to enjoy, such as going to the gym. She has been waking up in the middle of the night and has difficulty falling back to sleep.

During the interview, JO was initially anxious and irritable, but calmed down once she was able to engage in the conversation. She was cooperative and spontaneous in her responses to the questions.

C. *Past Psychiatric History*

When JO was 15 years old, she suffered from depression following the death of her father and took an overdose of unknown pills, which led to her being hospitalized for 3 days. Following discharge, she had some form of therapy, mostly via phone, and was prescribed medication (name unknown), but did not take it because she was afraid of potential side effects.

D. *Substance Use History*

JO reported that she smoked marijuana regularly for 5 years when she was with the twins' father so that they "would have something in common," but stopped when he left, except for one instance last summer when she smoked with her brother, as they were both very depressed following the death of their mother and he wanted her to smoke with him.

E. *Social and Developmental History*

1. *Education*: Dropped out of high school 3 months prior to graduation but obtained her GED certificate. Two years ago, she entered the police academy, but was expelled due to positive drug testing.
2. *Family Relationship, Social Network, and Abuse History*: JO was never married, had her first son at age 18 years old, and the twin boys at age 30

years old by a different father. She is not in contact with either father nor is she currently in a relationship. She has two brothers and two sisters; has a close relationship with one brother, but no contact with the other siblings.

JO reported that she was physically and sexually abused when she was 10 years old while placed in foster care. Additionally, she was raped by her cousin (reluctant to reveal detailed information) and was emotionally abused by the father of the twins.

3. *Employment Record*: JO has been working as a full-time medical assistant for the past 13 years. She claims to be a hard worker who rarely misses a day of work.
4. *Legal Record*: Denied having one.
5. *Religious Background*: Although raised Catholic, JO started to attend Baptist services with a friend to be with people following the mother's death, and was recently baptized in the Baptist Church.

F. *Family Psychiatric History*

JO reported that:
1. Her mother, maternal grandmother, and maternal aunt were diagnosed as "manic depressives," but was not clear whether any of them took medication except for the grandmother, who took "pills all her life."
2. A significant family history of substance use—both parents and 8 of her 11 maternal aunts and uncles were "drug addicts."
3. Oldest brother "emotionally disturbed," with a history of murdering someone years ago and being incarcerated for 13 years.
4. Other brother and sisters have no known psychiatric history.
5. One nephew diagnosed as schizophrenic.
6. Five-year-old twin boys, both diagnosed with ADHD and on Adderall.
7. Seventeen-year-old son: Two suicide attempts by taking pills and was admitted × 2 days after the last episode, which was last year.

G. *Medical History*

Last physical exam was 3 months ago. With her permission, the APMHN will obtain a copy of the results. JO reported that:
1. She was diagnosed with hypothyroidism and is currently on Synthroid (unclear the dosage). Other than that, no known physical illnesses are reported and no visually noticeable abnormalities noted.
2. No known allergies reported.
3. Weight: 154 lbs, gained 14 lbs within last month; height: 5'5"; BMI 26.

H. *Mental Status Examination*

1. *Appearance and Behavior*: The client was neatly dressed in her work uniform, good hygiene with hair neatly pulled back. She made good eye contact and was cooperative throughout the entire interview.
2. *Mood*: She stated that she felt "unorganized and drained." She appeared a little anxious at the beginning of the interview, but seemed to relax as time went on.

3. *Affect*: Her affect was appropriate to the current situation, and congruent to mood and thought contents.
4. *Thought Content and Process*: Speech was initially rapid, but after a few minutes, it slowed down to normal speed. Thought contents indicated no evidence of loose associations, tangential thought, thought blocking, or other signs of a formal thought disorder, including delusions or ideas of reference. Denied suicidal or homicidal ideations/intents/plans.
5. *Perceptual Disturbances*: She denies auditory, visual, or tactile hallucinations.
6. *Sensorium, Cognitive, and Intellectual Functioning*: JO was alert and oriented × 3. There was no evidence of gross cognitive dysfunction at any point during the interview. She demonstrated some insight and seemed to be motivated for treatment.

I. **Diagnosis and Treatment Plan**

1. **DSM-5 Diagnosis**: MDD, moderate.
2. **Rationale for Diagnostic Impression**: According to the DSM-5 (APA, 2013), to determine a diagnosis of MDD, the client must meet the following criteria, which JO meets as indicated by the bold symptom categories:

A. **Five (or more) of the following symptoms present nearly every day and at least one of the following 1 or 2 below criteria must be present:**
   1. **Depressed mood** most of the day:
      a. Subjective report of feelings of sadness, emptiness, hopelessness, or
      b. Observation made by others, such as tearful appearance.
         JO tears up easily, reports feelings of sadness and emptiness, and is isolating herself from her siblings.
   2. **Markedly diminished interest or pleasure** in all, or almost all, activities most of the day. JO reports that she no longer does things she used to enjoy.
   3. **Appetite-related significant weight change** (more than 5% of body weight loss or gain in a month when not dieting). JO has been eating more and has gained 14 lbs (10% of her weight) within the last 2 months.
   4. **Sleep disturbance** (insomnia or hypersomnia). JO has been waking up in the middle of the night and has difficulty falling back to sleep.
   5. Psychomotor agitation or retardation.
   6. **Fatigue or loss of energy.** JO feels that most days she doesn't have enough energy to do anything.
   7. Feelings of worthlessness or excessive or inappropriate guilt.
   8. Diminished ability to think or concentrate, or indecisiveness.
   9. Recurrent thoughts of death, recurrent suicidal ideation without a specific plan, or a suicide attempt or a specific plan for committing suicide.

B. **Duration: Five (or more) of the above signs or symptoms present during the same 2-week period.** JO reported that she has not been well since her mother's death a year ago, and her symptoms have been worse for the last 2 months.

C. *Impairment in Function: The symptoms cause clinically significant distress or impairment in social, occupational, or other important areas of functioning.* JO has been able to go to work regularly and perform her job functions; however, her relationship with family members, especially involving her twin sons and their father, has been highly stressful for her, as has been taking care of her children, who are also suffering from mental illnesses. Her weight gain due to overeating has led to her become overweight (BMI 26).

D. *Differential Diagnosis.* Careful consideration should be given to the delineation of normal sadness and grief from a major depressive episode. For example, bereavement may induce great suffering, but it does not typically induce an episode of MDD. In distinguishing grief from a major depressive episode, it is useful to consider that in grief, the predominant affect is feelings of emptiness and loss, while in a major depressive episode it is persistent depressed mood and the inability to anticipate happiness or pleasure.

Since the mother's death a year ago, in addition to feelings of sadness and emptiness, JO's depressed mood has been persistent. She is unable to experience pleasure, and has had prolonged sleep and appetite disturbances. Also, she has a history of depression, and multiple stress factors in her life exacerbate the symptoms of depression and anxiety.

E. *Diagnostic Recording.* In recording the name of a diagnosis, terms should be listed in the following order for clinical consistency:

1. Major depressive disorder: JO met five MDD symptom criteria.
2. Single or recurrent episode: JO had a previous episode of MDD.
3. Severity specifiers: JO met moderate severity based on the intensity of the symptoms as distressing but manageable, and that the symptoms have resulted in moderate impairment in social or occupational functioning.

Therefore, JO's diagnostic impression meets the criteria for a diagnosis of MDD, recurrent episode, moderate.

3. *Treatment Plan and Summary:*

Despite the diagnosis and one previous suicide attempt, JO is not considered to be a suicidal or homicidal risk, as evidenced by her denial of ideation/intent/plan, abstaining from substance use or abuse, genuinely seeking help for herself, and genuinely wanting to help her children. As JO is averse to medications to treat her depression with anxious distress, her treatment plan can be optimally served by a multifaceted approach, especially addressing the stressors in her life. It is believed that stress in those who have had multiple traumas can result in decreased activation of the prefrontal cortex; mindfulness therapy can help to activate this area and can be helpful in enhancing control over emotions (van der Kolk, 2006). Another consideration is to recommend that JO also join a bereavement support group, as such a group can help with difficulties with the grieving process. According to Zisook (2005), bereavement support groups provide "personal contact, information, an opportunity to share coping techniques, a sense of universality and belonging, increased self-worth, reinforcement for positive change, and an opportunity to help others." Interpersonal psychotherapy (IPT) might be useful, as JO has a number of responsibilities in her life and IPT is time limited and focused. With IPT, the therapist is active and proactive, while the change is the responsibility of the client (Barry, 2005). Lastly, JO's weight gain should be addressed, and it should be recommended that she follow up with her primary care provider to manage her hypothyroidism.

Section 3: Bipolar Disorders

Bipolar disorders are marked by severe mood swings between depression and elation, exhibited during distinct periods of abnormally and persistently elevated, expansive, or irritable mood, and accompanied with increased goal-directed activity or energy during an elation period. There are three major categories of bipolar disorders: (1) bipolar I: full manic or mixed episode, usually with a major depressive episode; (2) bipolar II: a major depressive episode and hypomanic episode (less intense than mania); and (3) cyclothymic disorder: a less severe type of bipolar disorder (Sadock & Sadock, 2010). According to the DSM-5 (APA, 2013), the estimated 12-month prevalence in the United States of bipolar I disorder is 0.6%, of bipolar II is 0.8%, and of cyclothymic disorder is 0.4–1%. Based on diagnostic interview data from the National Comorbidity Survey Replication (NCS-R), an estimated 4.4% of US adults experience bipolar disorder at some time in their lives (Information for Practice, 2012.). The effects of bipolar disorder can be far-reaching, both in the lives of clients and of their families, including work, school, relationships, finance, physical health, and many other aspects of everyday life. The most severe effect of bipolar disorder is suicide; 25–50% of people with bipolar disorder attempt suicide and 11% commit suicide (Tracy, 2012). Therefore, diagnoses included in this section are bipolar I and bipolar II, which will be used as examples of diagnostic assessment and evaluation, including treatment plans. The diagnostic criteria of bipolar disorders are modified from the DSM-5 (APA, 2013).

Diagnostic Criteria

The DSM-5 classifies bipolar disorders' diagnostic criteria presenting for manic and hypomanic episodes first, followed by criteria for bipolar I disorder and bipolar II disorder. The following description of the diagnostic criteria of both bipolar disorders does not present a major depressive episode, as that is described in the previous section.

DSM-5 Diagnostic Criteria: Manic Episode Modified

A. **Signs and Symptoms:**
   1. Elevated/expansive mood or irritable mood, and increased goal-directed activity or energy, and
   2. Presents three (or more) of the following symptoms (four if the mood is irritable) to a significant degree, which represents a noticeable change from usual behavior:
      a. Inflated self-esteem or grandiosity.
      b. Decreased need for sleep.
      c. More talkative than usual or pressure to keep talking.
      d. Flight of ideas or subjective experience that thoughts are racing.
      e. Distractibility, as reported or observed.
      f. Increased goal-directed activity or psychomotor agitation.
      g. Excessive involvement in activities that have a high potential for painful consequences (e.g., unrestrained buying sprees, foolish business investment, or sexual indiscretions).
B. **Duration:** Increased energy/activities presenting most of the day, nearly every day, for at least 1 week.
C. **Impairment in Function:** The mood disturbance is sufficiently severe to cause marked impairment in social or occupational function, or to necessitate hospitalization to prevent harm to self or others, or there are psychotic features.
D. **Differential Diagnosis:**
   1. Substance use/medication/other treatment-induced (e.g., drug abuse, antidepressant, electroconvulsive therapy) manic symptoms must be distinguished from bipolar I disorder.
   2. Criteria A–C constitute a manic episode and at least one manic episode is required for the diagnosis of bipolar disorder.

DSM-5 Diagnostic Criteria: Hypomanic Episode Modified

A. **Signs and Symptoms:**
   1. Elevated/expansive mood or irritable mood, and increased goal-directed activity or energy.
   2. Presents three (or more) of the following symptoms (four if the mood is irritable) to a significant degree, which represents a noticeable change from usual behavior:
      a. Inflated self-esteem or grandiosity.
      b. Decreased need for sleep.
      c. More talkative than usual or pressure to keep talking.
      d. Flight of ideas or subjective experience that thoughts are racing.
      e. Distractibility, as reported or observed.
      f. Increased goal-directed activity or psychomotor agitation.

g. Excessive involvement in activities that have a high potential for painful consequences (e.g., unrestrained buying sprees, foolish business investment, or sexual indiscretions).

B. **Duration:** Increased energy/activities presenting most of the day, nearly every day, for at least 4 consecutive days.

C. **Impairment in Function:**
1. The episode is not severe enough to cause marked impairment in social or occupational function or to necessitate hospitalization to prevent harm to self or others, nor are there psychotic features.
2. An equivocal change in functioning that is uncharacteristic of the individual when not symptomatic, but the changes in mood and functioning are observable by others.
3. The episode is not severe enough to cause marked impairment in social or occupational function nor to necessitate hospitalization.

DSM-5 Bipolar I Disorder Diagnostic Criteria Modified

A. For a diagnosis of bipolar I disorder, it is necessary to meet the criteria of at least one manic episode currently or in the past. Major depressive episodes are common in bipolar I disorder but are not required for its diagnosis.

B. Diagnostic recording: The diagnostic code for bipolar I disorder is based on the type of current or most recent episode, its severity (mild, moderate, or severe), and the presence of psychotic features, if indicated. In recording the name of a diagnosis, terms should be listed in the following order: Bipolar I disorder, type of episode (i.e., current or recent or remission), severity, psychotic features (if present), and specifiers (details of the descriptions of severity and type of episode can be found in the DSM-5, pages 126–127).

DSM-5 Bipolar II Disorder Diagnostic Criteria Modified

A. For a diagnosis of bipolar II disorder, it is necessary to have at least one hypomanic episode *and* at least one major depressive episode.

B. There has never been a manic episode.

C. The symptoms of depression or the unpredictability caused by frequent alternation between periods of depression or hypomania causes significant distress or impairment in social, occupational, or other important areas of functioning.

D. Diagnostic recording: Bipolar II disorder is coded with its status with current severity (mild, moderate, or severe), the presence of psychotic features, its course, and other specifiers. It should be recorded in the following order: Bipolar II disorder, most recent episode between hypomanic and depressed, in partial or full remission (if indicated), with specifiers between anxious distress and mixed features (details of the descriptions of severity, type of current and recent episodes, and specifiers can be found in the DSM-5, pages 134–135).

Differential Diagnosis:

A. Substance-/medication-induced hypomanic symptoms must be distinguished from bipolar disorders.
B. If there are psychotic features, the episode is, by definition, manic; therefore, it is bipolar I disorder.
C. There are no differences between the signs and symptoms of bipolar I and bipolar II disorders, but any past episodes of mania, the severity of functional impairment, and the duration of the episode are key to differentiating between either and cyclothymic disorder. See Table 2.8 for the differential diagnostic criteria among bipolar disorders.

Table 2.8 Differential Diagnostic Criteria among Bipolar Disorders

Type	Required Symptom Criteria	Minimum Symptom Duration	Functional Consequences as a Result of Bipolar Symptoms
Bipolar I	Minimum one manic episode	1 week	Marked impairment in social or occupational functioning, or necessitates hospitalization
Bipolar II	Minimum one hypomanic episode and one major depression	4 days	NOT severe enough to cause marked impairment in social or occupational functioning or to necessitate hospitalization
Cyclothymic	Both hypomanic and depressive periods without ever fulfilling the criteria for an episode of mania, hypomania, or major depression	Two years, with the hypomanic and depressive periods present at least half the time, and the individual having the symptoms for more than 2 months at a time	
Substance or medication induced	Medications that can induce manic symptoms are steroids and alpha interferon. Medications that can induce hypomanic episodes are antidepressants and electroconvulsive therapy		
Due to medical condition	Among the best-known medical conditions that can cause bipolar manic or hypomanic episodes are Cushing's disease, multiple sclerosis, stroke, or traumatic brain injuries		

Similar to what was discussed in Boxes 2.1 and 2.2, it is essential that APMHNs have a working knowledge of the neurobiological basis of bipolar disorder. Box 2.3 includes neurobiological theories of bipolar disorder, mainly focusing on the diagnostic symptom criteria of bipolar disorder and associated brain regions.

Box 2.3 Neurobiological Theories of Bipolar Disorder

In addition to understanding the DSM-5 diagnostic criteria for bipolar disorder, it is essential that APMHNs have a working knowledge of its neurobiological basis, especially the role of brain circuits and related symptom dimensions, in order to understand how psychotropic medications have been used in its treatment. Each diagnostic symptom for a manic or hypomanic episode is believed to be linked to alterations in neurotransmission within a certain brain region. Table 2.9 shows each brain region associated with a different constellation of symptoms.

Table 2.9 Diagnostic Symptom Criteria of Bipolar Disorder and Associated Brain Regions

Symptom Criteria of Manic Episode	Brain Regions
Elevated/expansive or irritable mood	Prefrontal cortex (PFC), amygdala (A)
Inflated self-esteem or grandiosity	Nucleus accumbens (NA), PFC
Decreased need for sleep	Thalamus (T), hypothalamus (HY)
More talkative or pressured speech	PFC
Flight of ideas or racing thoughts	NA, PFC
Distractible/concentration	PFC
Increased goal-directed activity or psychomotor agitation	Striatum (T)
Risk-taking behaviors	PFC

Source: Adapted from Stahl (2013).

Generally, the inefficient function in these brain circuits in mania may be the opposite of the malfunctioning neuronal circuits in the same key neurotransmitters (serotonin, norepinephrine, and dopamine) hypothesized for depression. There may also be activation in some overlapping and in some different brain regions that are activated in depression. Therefore, treatments for mania or hypomania either reduce or stabilize monoaminergic regulation of brain circuits associated with its symptoms (Stahl, 2013).

Interviewing Techniques in Assessment of Bipolar Disorders

As mentioned earlier, bipolar disorders are marked by severe mood swings between depression and hypomania or mania. Especially during the initial psychiatric interview of a client who presents with a chief complaint of depression, the depressed client may be too preoccupied with depressive symptoms to bring up a history of manic or hypomanic symptoms if not asked. Therefore, the APMHN should always inquire about prior manic or hypomanic symptoms during the initial interview of a depressed person.

The following sample questions would be helpful for the APMHN to elicit responses about the presence of any symptoms of mania or hypomania, and to differentiate between the types of bipolar disorder:

1. General question to target overall symptoms of bipolar disorder and its duration:
   a. *Is there a time in your life when you felt really super energized, did not need sleep, talked very fast, and did things like spending too much money or giving away valuables?*
   (This question would validate the DSM-5 symptom categories of bipolar disorder: inflated self-esteem or grandiosity, decreased need for sleep, more talkative than usual, and excessive involvement in activities that have a high potential for painful consequences. Following the response to this question, breaking down specific symptom-based short questions would be easier for the client to respond.)
   b. *Have there ever been several days or even weeks when you felt extremely energetic?*
   (This duration of symptoms would be helpful to differentiate between bipolar I disorder, for which symptoms last at least 1 week, and bipolar II disorder, for which symptoms last at least 4 days.)
   c. *Do you feel scattered, unproductive, and bothered by an unsettling sensation of bursts of low-grade energy so that you are just not yourself?*
   (This type of question would be helpful to elicit the symptoms of hypomania.)
   d. *Was there a time that things got so upsetting that you needed to be hospitalized?*
   (This question is to determine the severity of bipolar symptoms, since the hypomanic episode is not severe enough to necessitate hospitalization.)
2. Specific questions targeted to elicit each sign or symptom of bipolar disorder:
   a. *Was there a time in your life when you felt like you were on the top of the world and had special powers that other didn't?* (Grandiosity)
   b. *At some point in your life, did you experience that you didn't have to sleep for days because you had so much energy?* (Decreased need for sleep)
   c. *Do you recall starting to speak rapidly or did any of your friends remark that you are talking too fast?* (Hyperverbal)
   d. *Do you find your attention easily drawn to unimportant or irrelevant things?* (Distractibility)
   e. *Do you find that it's hard to keep track of your thoughts or do you experience racing thoughts?* (Flight of ideas)

    f. *Have you had any brilliant ideas or started several new activities lately?* (Increased goal-directed activity)

    g. *Have you ever done things that were out of character for you and that later you were embarrassed about, like spending too much money or giving valuables away?* (Indiscretion and recklessness)

The following is a case exemplar of an initial psychiatric evaluation that demonstrates how the diagnosis of bipolar disorder is determined, including the rationales and treatment plan for it.

Case Exemplar

The client's initials are BB.

A. *Identification, Chief Complaint, and Reason for Referral*

BB is a 47-year-old Caucasian female who presented with the chief complaint, "I just can't sleep anymore and my primary care doctor sent me to this clinic for a psychiatric evaluation."

B. *History of Present Illness*

BB reported that since her 25-year-old son was diagnosed with brain cancer 9 months ago, she has been extremely irritable and easily agitated: "Nobody can talk to me—I bite their heads off! I don't want to be around anybody; they all get on my nerves. I've gotten to the point that I just keep things to myself. I don't go anywhere, and I don't do anything. My mother tries to get me to come out of my room, but I just want to stay in bed and watch TV all day." BB further elaborated that she got fired from her job as a retail sales associate 2 months ago following an altercation with her supervisor. Usually, she could deal with the supervisor's attitude, but that day she just snapped and threw everything out the window, which led to her termination. After that, she was not able to pay her rent and ended up moving into her mother's place last month. Her inability to support herself contributes to BB's feelings of worthlessness and social isolation. She feels no desire to look for a job and to get her life together. When BB went to see her primary care doctor for a routine check-up, she was told to get help from a mental health clinic. She agreed to come to the clinic. Initial psychiatric evaluation revealed low mood, increased levels of agitation, anhedonia, and difficulty concentrating. She reported having thoughts recently of "just not being here," but denies suicide ideation/intent/plans. BB also suffers from decreased motivation, low energy, insomnia, feelings of worthlessness, agitation, and irritability.

C. *Past Psychiatric History*

BB denied a history of psychotic symptoms and psychiatric hospitalization, and reported no past history of suicidal attempts. Assessment revealed no history of manic episodes, but careful inquiry exposed hypomanic episodes, beginning in her early 20s, during which BB described herself as unusually productive, creative, and sociable, and "able to go all day and night without much sleep." During these episodes, BB reported getting two speeding tickets and going on shopping sprees, stating that she got into trouble with overdrawn credit cards a few times. BB reported intermittent treatment of depressive symptoms since her early 20s, typically prescribed by her primary care provider, but on occasion by her gynecologist. She has either been treated with monotherapy antidepressants or a combination of antidepressants and benzodiazepine. She stated that she received both of her traffic citations while on fluoxetine therapy. While exploring her past history, BB stated that she realized most of her spending sprees occurred during antidepressant treatment. Her medication treatment for depression includes trials of sertraline, citalopram, venlafaxine XR, and bupropion. BB reported modest improvement of depressive mood with these antidepressants, and at times was treated with diazepam or lorazepam for her anxiety. BB has also received trazodone for insomnia, which in the past has helped her to sleep better. She stated that she has not been compliant with the prescribed medications for longer than 5 or 6 months because the medications either did not seem to help her depression or she felt so good that she believed she was cured. BB last received treatment for her mood symptoms 3 years ago.

D. *Substance Use History*

BB reported a history of using roughly one to two grams of marijuana two to three times weekly to help her sleep. Her last marijuana use was last night before she went to sleep. She denied drinking alcohol or using other drugs, including tobacco.

E. *Social and Developmental History*

BB is currently residing with her mother, who is supportive and available to her, especially when she is in "trouble," referring to her mood swings. However, BB has alienated herself from other relatives and friends due to those frequent mood swings. She claims that she wants to feel better so that she can accomplish her dream of owning her own business.

1. *Education*: BB dropped out of high school in eleventh grade, and later obtained her GED certificate.
2. *Family Relationship, Social Network, and Abuse History*: BB was born in Long Island, New York, and is the older child of two siblings. She recalls growing up in a chaotic family, most of whom suffered some sort of mental illness and substance use (see the family psychiatric history). She was married to an alcoholic man for 5 years and had one son. Currently, she resides with her mother after being fired from her job. BB is close to the mother, who has been supportive of her throughout her

life. BB claimed that she has been very close to her son and his illness was the main reason why she has been "falling apart." She denied any history of trauma, such as exposure to violence or sexual or physical abuse during her childhood.

3. *Employment Record*: BB has had various occupations, mostly in retail clothing stores as a retail sales associate, as she was known to be socially pleasant and good with customers. However, each employment did not last more than a year due to her mood swings and frequent absenteeism.

4. *Legal Records*: BB denies any problem with the law and denies any criminal records other than traffic tickets.

F. *Family Psychiatric History*

BB's family has a significant mental illness and substance use history:

1. Mental illness:
   - Maternal grandmother and sister—bipolar disorder.
   - Mother—anxiety disorder.
   - Son—attention deficit hyperactivity disorder and depression.
2. Substance use:
   - Maternal grandmother, both paternal grandparents—tobacco.
   - Maternal grandmother, both grandfathers, father, mother, sister, and son—alcohol.
   - Father, brother, and son—cannabis.
   - Son—methamphetamine.

G. *Medical History and Review of System*

BB reported:

1. Current medical conditions and related treatments as following:
   - Hypothyroidism, treated with levothyroxine 0.75 mg daily.
   - Osteoarthritis, treated with celecoxib 200 mg daily.
   - Hypertension, treated with lisinopril 10 mg daily, hydrochlorothiazide 12.5 mg daily.
2. Past medical history:
   - A total hysterectomy at age 37, secondary to menorrhagia related to fibroid tumors.
   - A tonsillectomy at age 2, secondary to recurrent tonsillitis and ear infections.
3. Allergic to penicillin and quinolones (urticaria with each).
4. Vital signs: BP: 120/80; HR: 70; RR: 20; Temp: 98 F; Ht: 5'5"; Wt: 125 lbs; BMI: 21.
5. Review of systems showed no significant observable overall physical abnormalities.

H. *Mental Status Examination*

1. *Appearance and Behavior*: BB appears to be the stated age; general appearance is well-kept with good personal hygiene; overall behavior is cooperative with good eye contact during the interview; speech fluent, linear, logical, and coherent.
2. *Mood*: Anxious, labile varying between sad and angry.
3. *Affect*: Irritable, tearful, and withdrawn.
4. *Thought Content and Process*: No evidence of delusions, denied suicidal ideations/intent/plans, no abnormality in thought content and thought process present.
5. *Perceptional Disturbances*: Denied auditory, visual, and tactile hallucinations.
6. *Sensorium, Cognitive, and Intellectual Functioning*: BB is alert and oriented × 3. Attention span and concentration are intact, intellectual functioning is on average level.

I. *Diagnosis and Treatment Plan*

1. **DSM-5 Diagnosis:** BB's diagnosis is recorded as bipolar II disorder, moderate, most recent episode of depression, anxious distress (details of the descriptions of severity, type of current and recent episodes, and specifiers can be found in the DSM-5, pages 149–154).
2. **Rationale for Diagnostic Impression:** According to the DSM-5 (APA, 2013), to diagnose bipolar II disorder, the following criteria must be present, either in the past or currently. BB met these criteria, as indicated by the bold symptom categories:

A. *At least one hypomanic episode and at least one major depressive episode must be present either in the past or currently. Below is a description of BB's symptom manifestations, which meet Criteria 1 and 2:*

1. *At least one hypomanic episode.* BB experienced a hypomanic episode in the past, with increased energy/activities presenting most of the day, nearly every day, lasting at least 4 consecutive days, as evidenced by three self-reported symptoms of:
   a. *Increased goal-directed activity or energy* evidenced by BB's self-report of "unusually productive, creative, sociable."
   b. *Decreased need for sleep* evidenced by BB's self-report of "able to go all day and night on 3 hours sleep."
   c. *Excessive involvement in activities that have a high potential for painful consequences* evidenced by BB's self-report of "enjoys shopping and has gotten into trouble with credit cards a few times."
2. *At least one major depressive episode.* BB reported a major depressive episode in the past and present, with seven symptoms (see the quotation next to each depressive symptom criterion) from the DSM-5's major depressive symptom criteria present during the same 2-week period (requires a minimum of five symptoms), and representing a change from previous functioning:

a. *Depressed mood most of the day.* "low mood."
b. *Markedly diminished interest or pleasure in all, or almost all, activities most of the day.* "I've gotten to where I just keep to myself. I don't go anywhere, and I don't do anything."
c. *Feelings of worthlessness or excessive or inappropriate guilt.* "feelings of worthlessness and social isolation."
d. *Psychomotor agitation.* "increased levels of anxiety, agitation, and irritability."
e. *Diminished ability to think or concentrate, or indecisiveness.* "difficulty concentrating."
f. *Fatigue or loss of energy.* "low energy."
g. *Sleep disturbance.* "insomnia."

B. *There has never been a manic episode.* BB reported that she never had a manic episode in her life.

C. *The symptoms of depression or the unpredictability caused by frequent alternation between periods of depression and hypomania causes significant distress or impairment in social and/or occupational functioning.* BB reported her inability to keep a job, financial constraints, social isolation, and poor interpersonal relationships.

3. *Summary and Treatment Plan*: In this section, a brief summary is added for the APMHN to elaborate when diagnosing clients presenting with a common disorder:

- *Summary*: BB suffers from bipolar disorder II, which started in her 20s, subjectively experienced as "mood swings," but was misdiagnosed as depression since BB only reported depressed mood to her healthcare providers. Approximately 60% of patients with bipolar disorder who present with depressive symptoms are misdiagnosed as having recurrent depression (Phillips & Kupfer, 2013), which can lead to inappropriate treatments, with worsening of symptoms. Unfortunately, BB was treated with antidepressants by nonpsychiatric specialists, which might have precipitated antidepressant-induced hypomanic or manic episodes. Ultimately, unchecked hypomanic symptoms led to risky behaviors, through which BB sustained severe damage to relationships, careers, and finances.

- *Treatment plan*: Explain to the client and the family the appropriate treatment plan, including the accurate diagnosis following psychiatric evaluation by the APMHN, adequate treatment options based on the evidence, and the client treatment-related preferences:
  - *Level of care*: Outpatient clinic. Currently, BB presents no imminent danger to self or others, but is willing to accept the recommended treatment in the outpatient mental health clinic.
  - *Screening for bipolar disorder*: A rigorous screening for a client who presents a potential diagnosis of bipolar disorder with validated screening instruments (e.g., mood disorder questionnaire, bipolar spectrum diagnostic scale, rapid mood screener).

- *Psychopharmacological treatment*: Guidelines for pharmaco-therapy for bipolar depression have been developed through a collaboration between the Canadian Network for Mood and Anxiety Treatments and the International Society for Bipolar Disorders (Yatham et al., 2018). Since BB is diagnosed with "bipolar II disorder, moderate, most recent episode of depression, anxious distress," medication options based on the evidence, using the guidelines and BB's medication-related preferences, could be explored and a decision made as to appropriate psychopharmacological treatment.

Section 4: Anxiety Disorders

Anxiety disorders are classified in the DSM-5 as 11 distinct diagnostic disorders. They can be viewed as a group of related mental disorders that share features of excessive fear and anxiety, as well as related behavioral disturbances. Anxiety disorders make up the most common group of psychiatric disorders, with a 12-month prevalence rate of approximately 17% in the United States. Phobia is the most common disorder, with a lifetime prevalence of 10% and an average age onset of late 20s, followed by generalized anxiety disorder, with a lifetime prevalence of 3–8% and an average onset of early adulthood (Sadock et al., 2019).

However, most anxiety disorders develop in childhood, and tend to persist if not treated. As with depressive disorders, women are twice as likely as men to be affected (APA, 2013). Signs and symptoms manifest both psychologically and physically. Psychological symptoms are feelings of dread, hypervigilance, and difficulty concentrating, while physical symptoms involve a hyperactive autonomic nervous system, which manifests as tachycardia, sweating, dry mouth, flushing, and other somatic complaints, such as shortness of breath (SOB) and trembling (Sadock et al., 2019). Due to the nature of this disorder's common concurrent symptom manifestations, it is especially important that the APMHN understands and respects the client's perspective and experience, and that they rule out other potential medical illnesses, to make a proper diagnosis and treatment plan. Conducting a psychiatric evaluation of a client presenting with symptoms of anxiety disorder requires a skillful diagnostic interview to obtain accurate information while building a rapport and therapeutic alliance with the client. The goal of this approach is to improve client engagement, client knowledge of diagnosis and treatment options, and collaborative decision-making with the APMHN about treatment.

Table 2.10 lists the specific anxiety disorders in the DSM-5, differentiated by type, followed by brief descriptions.

In addition to understanding the DSM-5 diagnostic criteria for anxiety disorders, it is essential that APMHNs have a working knowledge of their neurobiological basis, especially the role of brain circuits and related symptom dimensions,

Table 2.10 Anxiety Disorder Diagnostic Classification

Diagnosis Classification	Specific Diagnosis	Type of Objects or Situation, and/or Essential Feature of Each Anxiety Disorder
Specific phobia	Acrophobia	Fear of heights
	Agoraphobia	Fear of open places
	Ailurophobia	Fear of cats
	Claustrophobia	Fear of closed spaces
	Cynophobia	Fear of dogs
	Hydrophobia	Fear of water
	Mysophobia	Fear of dirt and germs
	Pyrophobia	Fear of fire
	Xenophobia	Fear of strangers
	Zoophobia	Fear of animals
DSM-5 Classification of Anxiety Disorders		
Agoraphobia	Intense fear or anxiety triggered by the real or anticipated exposure to a wide range of situations (e.g., using public transportation, being in open spaces, enclosed places, in crowds, or outside of the home alone); symptom severity is a strong determinant of disability; more than one-third of agoraphobic clients are completely homebound and unable to work	
Social anxiety disorder	Irrational fear of public situations (e.g., speaking in public, eating in public, using public bathrooms)	
Panic disorder	Characterized by spontaneous panic attacks, which may evolve in stages: subclinical attacks, full panic attacks, anticipatory anxiety, or phobic avoidance of specific situations; this disorder may occur alone or be associated with agoraphobia	
Generalized anxiety disorder	Involves excessive worry about everyday life circumstances, events, or conflicts; symptoms may fluctuate and overlap with other medical and psychiatric disorders, such as depressive and other anxiety disorders	
Substance-/medication-induced anxiety disorder	A wide range of substances can cause anxiety symptoms that are often associated with intoxication or withdrawal states	
Anxiety disorder due to another medical condition	A wide range of medical conditions can cause anxiety symptoms; also, a number of medical conditions are known to include anxiety as a symptomatic manifestation, such as hyperthyroidism, hypoglycemia, angina pectoris/myocardial infarction, asthma, vitamin B12 deficiency, and neoplasms	
Anxiety disorders that differ from developmental disorders		
Selective mutism	Inability to speak in certain social situations despite the ability to speak in other circumstances	
Separational anxiety disorder	Developmentally inappropriate and excessive fear and anxiety over separation from home or loved ones	

Source: Adapted from Sadock et al. (2019).

in order to understand how psychotropic medications have been used in treatment. Box 2.4 summarizes the neurobiological theories of anxiety disorders.

Box 2.4 Neurobiological Theories of Anxiety Disorders

Although there are different diagnostic criteria for different anxiety disorders, they all have overlapping symptoms of anxiety and fear, coupled with worry. Hypothetically, anxiety and fear symptoms are regulated by an amygdala-centered circuit, while worry is regulated by a cortico-striato-thalamo-cortical (CTSC) circuit. However, what differentiates one anxiety disorder from another may not be the anatomical localization or the neurotransmitters regulating fear and worry, but the specific nature of the malfunctioning within the same circuits.

Table 2.11 Anxiety Disorder–Associated Symptoms Malfunctioning in Brain Regions and Circuits

Core symptom of anxiety: Fear	*Overactivation of amygdala circuit reciprocal or activating connection with*
Panic and phobia	• Anterior cingulate cortex/-orbitofrontal cortex
Avoidance; motor response	• Periaqueductal gray
Endocrine output of fear; increased cortisol release	• Hypothalamic–pituitary–adrenal (HPA) axis
Breathing output; shortness of breath	• Parabrachial nucleus (PBN)
Autonomic output of fear; increased heart beat and blood pressure	• Locus coeruleus
Re-experiencing; feature of PTSD	• Hippocampus (storage of traumatic memories)
Linking "fear" to amygdala circuits to neurotransmitters and voltage-gated iron channels	• Malfunctioning of amygdala-centered circuits which are regulated by neurotransmitters (serotonin, GABA, glutamate, norepinephrine) and voltage-gated iron channels
Core symptom of anxiety: **Worry**	Malfunction of **CTSC** circuit
Worry; anxious misery, apprehensive expectations, catastrophic thinking, ruminations, and obsessions	• Overactivation of the CTSC circuit ending in the dorsolateral prefrontal cortex
Linking "worry" to CTSC circuits to neurotransmitters and voltage-gated iron channels	• Malfunctioning of CTSC circuits which are regulated by neurotransmitters (serotonin, dopamine, GABA, glutamate, norepinephrine) and voltage-gated iron channels

Source: Adapted from Stahl (2013).

For example, in generalized anxiety disorder, malfunctioning in the amygdala and cortico-striato-thalamo-cortical circuits is persistent and unremitting, yet not severe, while in panic disorder, the same malfunctioning is intermittent but catastrophic in an unexpected manner, and in social anxiety disorder it is intermittent but catastrophic in an expected manner. In post-traumatic stress disorder (PTSD), circuit malfunctioning may be both traumatic in origin and conditioned (Stahl, 2013). For APMHNs to treat their clients with anxiety disorders, it is essential that they understand how the GABA, other neurotransmitters, and iron channels regulate brain circuits. Table 2.11 presents malfunctioning in brain regions and circuits for different symptoms of anxiety disorders.

Furthermore, as a wide range of medical conditions either cause anxiety symptoms or include anxiety as one of several symptoms, when an APMHN evaluates a client with a probable anxiety disorder, it is useful to rule out a potential medical etiology of anxiety during the diagnostic evaluation (Table 2.12).

Table 2.12 Differential Diagnosis of Common Medical Conditions Mimicking Anxiety

Common Medical Conditions	Common Symptoms	Rule Out with Test/Intervention
Angina pectoris/ myocardial infarction (MI)	Crushing chest pain, usually associated with angina/MI	Electrocardiogram with ST depression in angina; cardiac enzymes in MI
Hyperventilation syndrome	Rapid and deep respirations, circumoral pallor, carpopedal spasm	Respond to rebreathing in paper bag
Hypoglycemia	Signs of diabetes mellitus; polyuria, polydipsia, polyphagia	Fasting blood sugar usually under 50 mg/dL
Hyperthyroidism	Anxiety, restlessness, and irritability	Thyroid function tests; decreased thyroid stimulating hormone (TSH), but elevated triiodothyronine (T3), thyroxine (T4)

Source: Adapted from Sadock et al. (2019).

In this section, generalized anxiety disorder (GAD) is selected as an example of a presenting anxiety disorder, as it represents the classic condition in this group of disorders. GAD is known to be associated with significant disability and distress, and most noninstitutionalized adults with the disorder are moderately to seriously disabled (APA, 2013).

Diagnostic Criteria

DSM-5 GAD Diagnostic Criteria Modified

A. **Signs and Symptoms:** Excessive anxiety and worry about a number of events or activities, such as work or school performance. The anxiety and worry are associated with three (or more) of the following six symptoms:
   1. Restlessness or feeling keyed up or on edge.
   2. Being easily fatigued.
   3. Difficulty concentrating or mind going blank.
   4. Irritability.
   5. Muscle tension.
   6. Sleep disturbance.
B. **Duration:** Symptoms occurring more days than not for at least 6 months.
C. **Impairment in Function:** The symptoms cause clinically significant distress or impairment in social, occupational, or other important areas of functioning.
D. **Differential Diagnosis:**
   1. The symptoms are not attributable to the physiological effects of a substance (e.g., drug use, adverse reaction of medication) or other medical condition (e.g., hyperthyroidism, hypoglycemia).
   2. The disturbance is not better explained by other mental disorders.
   3. Symptoms of autonomic hyperarousal (e.g., accelerated heart rate, shortness of breath, dizziness) are less prominent in GAD than in other anxiety disorders.

Interviewing Techniques in Assessment of GAD

The following questions are examples for the APMHN to consider when evaluating a client's presenting symptoms to formulate a final diagnosis, based on the DSM-5 symptom criteria of GAD:

1. *Would you describe yourself as a chronic worrier or do you hear from others that you are always worrying about things? (DSM-5 symptom criteria: "Excessive anxiety and worry about a number of events or activities, such as work or school performance").*
2. *If you do, how often and how long has this been going on? (DSM-5 symptom criteria: "Symptoms occurring more days than not for at least 6 months").*
3. *Over the past few months of worrying, have you noticed that you have been jittery, on edge, or irritable? (DSM-5 symptom criteria: "Restlessness or feeling keyed up or on edge," "Irritability").*
4. *Do you often experience tension in your head and neck or any other parts of your body? (DSM-5 symptom criteria: "Muscle tension").*
5. *What has your sleep been like? (DSM-5 symptom criteria: "Sleep disturbance").*

6. *Do you experience difficulty in concentrating on tasks because your mind often goes blank? (DSM-5 symptom criteria: "Difficulty concentrating or mind going blank").*

7. *Do you find yourself being tired easily? (DSM-5 symptom criteria: "Being easily fatigued").*

8. *Some people are worriers but they can usually handle it. Other people are such severe worriers that they find that worrying gets in the way of their life or paralyzes them. Which one sounds more like you? (DSM-5 symptom criteria: "The symptoms cause clinically significant distress or impairment in social, occupational, or other important areas of functioning").*

9. *How would you describe what your typical day is like? (Asking about the client's typical day can open up a cache of diagnostically rich data that may help the APMHN to grasp an overall picture of the client's life).*

The following is a case exemplar of an initial psychiatric evaluation, including how the diagnosis of GAD is determined, with a proposed treatment plan and rationales.

Case Exemplar

The client's initials are Ms. M.

A. *Identification, Chief Complaint, and Reason for Referral*

Ms. M is a 49-year-old Caucasian female who works as an account executive and was referred to the outpatient clinic by her primary care provider for psychiatric evaluation and treatment. Her chief complaint is, "I've dealt with anxiety most of my life, but lately it has taken control of my life."

B. *History of the Present Illness*

Ms. M reported that over the past 7 months following her promotion to supervisor at her job, she has noticed that every little thing is causing her to be overly anxious. Her wife has also noticed this change in her behavior and has been doing her best to take on extra responsibilities in the home to give Ms. M a break. Ms. M has been dealing with considerable amounts of anxiety and worry almost every day. She complained that her mind was consumed by constant worrying, ruminating about things she felt she might have forgotten to do throughout the day, unable to focus, with poor concentration at work. Recently, she has found that many of her work projects have become overwhelming and are causing her excessive stress, and that she has had trouble completing them on time. In addition, she complained of waves of nervousness and trembling, with a mild degree of shortness of breath and heart palpitations. She also reported having sleep problems, usually tossing and turning for 30–90 minutes before falling asleep. Not getting adequate sleep, Ms. M reported restlessness and fatigue throughout the day. Ms. M is now concerned that she has been constantly irritable around her wife, which has been affecting her marriage.

C. *Past Psychiatric History*

Ms. M reports no past history of psychiatric treatments, either outpatient or inpatient in a hospital setting, and no prior diagnosed psychiatric symptoms before the onset of the current episode. However, she admitted that she has always been a worrier and others, like her wife and close friends, have told her that she worries about everything all the time.

D. *Substance Use History*

Ms. M denies any use of alcohol, cocaine, opiates, amphetamines, marijuana, nicotine, or any other illicit drugs.

E. *Social and Developmental History*

1. *Education*: Completion of MBA program with honors.
2. *Family Relationship, Social Network, and Abuse History*: Lives with wife and two teenage children (14-year-old girl and 16-year-old boy). Has not maintained relationships with friends due to her excessive anxiety since promotion to supervisor at her current job. No history of abuse.
3. *Legal Records*: Ms. M has no history of arrest or any pending legal case.
4. *Religious Background*: Christian.

F. *Family History*

Ms. M claimed that there was no history of psychiatric illness among family and relatives.

G. *Medical History and Review of Systems*: The APMHN conducted a full physical examination.

1. Vital signs: B/P: 110/70; HR: 98; R/R: 18; Temp: 98.6 F; Ht: 5'4"; Wt: 119 lbs.
2. General: No acute distress (NAD), alert, awake, and oriented × 4 (AAO × 4) to name, place, time, purpose, well-developed and well-nourished (WDWN) white female.
3. Head, eyes, ears, nose, throat (HEENT): Normocephalic atraumatic (NCAT), mucous membranes moist (MMM), extraocular muscles intact (EOMI), pupils equally round and reactive to light and accommodation bilaterally (PERRLA), bilateral tympanic membrane (b/l TM) intact and reactive to light, bilateral sclera anicteric, no conjunctival injection.
4. Cardiovascular (CV): Regular rate and rhythm (RRR), S1S2 normal, no chest pain, but reported occasional palpitations during anxiety episodes.
5. Pulmonary: Clear to auscultation bilaterally (CTAB), no rales/rhonchi/wheezes (R/R/W), no egophany, no tactice fremitus, normal percussion, mild degree of shortness of breath during anxiety episodes.

6. Gastrointestinal (GI): Normal bowel sound (BS) throughout four quadrants, non-distended, non-tender, no nausea, vomiting, or diarrhea.
7. Genitourinary (GU): No gynecological or urological issues reported.
8. Skin: Intact, no rashes, erythema, or lesions.
9. Neurologic: Cranial nerves II to XII intact.
10. Musculoskeletal: Normal range of motion (ROM), no complaint of joint pain, stiffness, or swelling, and normal gait.
11. Allergies: No known allergies reported.

H. *Mental Status Examination*

1. *Appearance and Behavior*: The client was a casually dressed, 49-year-old Caucasian woman, who appeared to be the stated age. She was cooperative, made good eye contact with the interviewer throughout the entire interview, but irritable, with frequent handwringing and shifting of her legs.
2. *Mood*: Anxious.
3. *Affect*: Irritable, mildly tense, and mood congruent.
4. *Thought Content and Process*: Speech was fluent, with normal tone and volume, linear and goal directed, and coherent. Thought contents indicated no evidence of loose associations, tangential thought, thought blocking, or other signs of a formal thought disorder, including delusions or ideas of reference. Denied suicidal or homicidal ideations/intents/plans.
5. *Perceptual Disturbances*: Denied any forms of perceptual disturbances, including auditory, visual, or tactile hallucinations.
6. *Sensorium, Cognitive, and Intellectual Functioning*: Alert and oriented × 4. There was no evidence of gross cognitive dysfunction at any point during the interview. She acknowledged poor concentration and difficulty focusing on her daily tasks due to her anxiety, and is motivated for treatment.

I. *Diagnostic Screens and Laboratory Tests*

In this section, an example that demonstrates evidence-based practice is added as a result of the final diagnostic screening:
1. Generalized Anxiety Disorder 7-item (GAD-7) scale was used to assess the severity of Ms. M's anxiety symptoms. This tool assists in supporting a diagnosis of GAD. Ms. M scored a 12; a score above 10 is indicative of moderate anxiety and warrants further assessment (Spitzer et al., 2006).
2. The following laboratory tests were ordered to rule out common medical conditions mimicking anxiety: complete blood count (CBC) w/differential; basic metabolic panel (BMP); liver function test (LFT); urine tox; hormone panel: thyroid stimulating hormone (TSH), T3, T4, estradiol, follicle stimulating hormone (FSH), luteinizing hormone (LH) to assess kidney and liver functioning, as well as to rule out any organic cause for the symptoms of anxiety, such as thyroid dysfunction/menopause or illicit drug use (McCance & Huether, 2018).

J. *Diagnosis and Treatment Plan*

1. *DSM-5 Diagnosis*: GAD, moderate.
2. *Rationale for Diagnostic Impression*: According to the DSM-5 (APA, 2013), the following criteria must be present in order to diagnose GAD. Ms. M meets those criteria, as indicated by the bold symptom categories A–E:

A. *Excessive anxiety and worry* (apprehensive expectation), occurring more days than not for at least 6 months. Ms. M has reported that over the past 7 months, she has noticed that every little thing is causing her to be overly anxious and that she has been dealing with considerable amounts of anxiety and worry almost every day.

B. *The individual finds it difficult to control the worry.* Ms. M's chief complaint at the time of evaluation was, "I've dealt with anxiety most of my life but lately it has taken control of my life."

C. *The anxiety and worry are associated with three or more of the following symptoms:*
   1. *Restlessness or feeling keyed up or on edge*: Ms. M complained of waves of nervousness and trembling, with shortness of breath and heart palpitations.
   2. *Being easily fatigued*: Ms. M complained of feeling tired easily.
   3. *Difficulty concentrating or mind going blank*: She complained that her mind was consumed by constant worrying, ruminating about things she felt she might have forgotten to do throughout the day, unable to focus, with poor concentration at work.
   4. *Irritability*: She reported that she frequently became restless and irritable.
   5. *Muscle tension*: She did not complain of muscle tension.
   6. *Sleep disturbance*: She reported having sleep problems, usually tossing and turning for 30–90 minutes before falling asleep. Not getting adequate sleep.

D. *Social, occupational, functional impairment.* Recently, she has found that many of her work projects have become overwhelming and cause her excessive stress, and that she has had trouble completing them on time. Ms. M is also concerned that she has been constantly irritable around her wife, which has been affecting her marriage.

E. *Differential diagnosis: Substance/medication induced or related to medical conditions.* Ms. M denied substance use and reported no obvious common medical conditions mimicking anxiety.

The APMHN concluded that Ms. M met the DSM-5 GAD diagnostic criteria as shown by the above descriptions of the symptom presentations.

3. *Treatment Plan*: Explain to Ms. M the proposed treatment plan, including the diagnosis and treatment options, and ask about her treatment-related preferences:

- Psychotherapy (e.g., cognitive behavioral therapy [CBT], mindfulness-based stress reduction).
- Psychopharmacology (e.g., selective serotonin reuptake inhibitor [SSRI], selective norepinephrine reuptake inhibitor [SNRI], benzodiazepine).

The following document is an example of a client's psychiatric evaluation, including a treatment plan prepared to send to the referring clinician, as sometimes the referring clinician requests the narrative summary rather than the formal psychiatric evaluation.

Ms. M is a 49-year-old Caucasian female who works as an account executive who you referred to the outpatient clinic for psychiatric evaluation and treatment. The patient described her anxiety as being out of control, impairing her functioning at work and home, causing her irritability, fatigue, and insomnia. Moreover, she mentioned palpitations and shortness of breath on occasion during episodes of intense anxiety. Ms. M was also concerned that her anxiety is interfering with her marriage. She has no prior psychiatric treatment history regarding herself or her immediate family members. In addition, Ms. M denies any use of illicit drugs, herbal supplements, tobacco products, or caffeine. She reported no prior psychiatric treatment and currently indicated no imminent danger to herself or others.

A comprehensive psychiatric evaluation concluded, based on the patient's symptomology, that she met the diagnostic criteria for generalized anxiety disorder, moderate, based on the Generalized Anxiety Disorder 7-item scale. Goals and interventions were discussed and Ms. M verbalized understanding. A consult for psychotherapy, such as cognitive behavioral therapy or mindfulness-based stress reduction, will assist Ms. M in managing and becoming aware of triggers for her anxiety. Ms. M will be started on 37.5 mg venlafaxine XR, which is a selective norepinephrine reuptake inhibitor, once daily for 7 days, and will then increase to 75 mg daily. Until symptoms improve, can increase dosage by 75 mg every 3 to 4 weeks, not to exceed 225 mg/day for the treatment of GAD. As Ms. M does not have a history of illicit drug use, lorazepam 0.25 mg three times daily will be prescribed, with the last dose before bedtime. No prior illicit drug use indicates a lower possibility of Ms. M developing habituation of benzodiazepines. However, lorazepam will be discontinued within 6 weeks to prevent her from developing physiological dependence, pending evaluation at the time. Efficacy of the medications taking at least 2–4 weeks to work and of tolerability, including side effects of venlafaxine XR, were discussed, as well as potential dependency on benzodiazepine use. If venlafaxine XR is not well tolerated, will consider selective serotonin reuptake inhibitor such as paroxetine, which has been shown to be effective in treating GAD. Ms. M verbalized understanding and is in agreement with the treatment plan. She is scheduled for re-evaluation in 2 weeks.

Section 5: Obsessive-Compulsive and Related Disorders

Obsessive-compulsive disorder (OCD) is characterized by the presence of (1) obsessions, which are recurrent, persistent, and intrusive thoughts, urges, or images; and (2) compulsions, which are repetitive behaviors or mental acts that an individual feels driven to perform in response to an obsession or according to rules that must be applied rigidly. A person with OCD may have an obsession, a compulsion, or both (APA, 2013). There are a variety of OCD-related disorders, such as body dysmorphic disorder, hoarding disorder, trichotillomania (hair pulling), and excoriation disorder (skin picking). OCD is the fourth most common psychiatric disorder, and the lifetime prevalence of OCD in the general US population is estimated at 1–3%. The mean age of onset is approximately 20 years, and among adults, women are affected at a slightly higher rate than are men. Approximately 50–70% of clients with OCD have a sudden onset of symptoms following a stressful event, such as the death of a loved one, a serious illness, or a sexual problem (Sadock et al., 2019). Many OCD clients have full insight that their behaviors are senseless and excessive.

Table 2.13 presents the variety of obsessions and their related compulsions.

In this section, obsessive-compulsive disorder is selected as an example of a presenting OCD-related disorder, as it represents the classic condition in this group of disorders.

Table 2.13 Symptom Patterns of Obsessions and Compulsions

Patterns of Obsession	*Related Compulsions*	*Comments*
Contamination (e.g., germs)	Washing, cleaning, and/ or avoiding presumably contaminated objects	The most common pattern of OCD
Pathologic doubt (e.g., door lock)	Repetitive checking	The second most common pattern of OCD
Intrusive thoughts (e.g., suicidal, aggressive, sexual, religious thoughts)	Intrusive thoughts may or may not be accompanied by compulsive behaviors	The third most common pattern of OCD; risk of potential harm to self or others should be evaluated carefully
Symmetry (e.g., precision)	Repeating words silently, ordering, counting	The fourth most common pattern of OCD
Preoccupation with perceived defects or flaws in physical appearance	Mirror checking, excessive grooming, seeking reassurance in response to physical appearance	DSM-5 diagnosis: Body dysmorphic disorder
Persistent difficulty discarding or parting with possessions, regardless of their value	Hoarding	DSM-5 diagnosis: Hoarding disorder
Recurrent urge of pulling out one's hair, resulting in hair loss	Hair pulling	DSM-5 diagnosis: Trichotillomania
Recurrent urge of picking skin, resulting in skin lesions	Skin picking	DSM-5 diagnosis: Excoriation disorder

Source: Partially adapted from Sadock et al. (2019).

Diagnostic Criteria

DSM-5 OCD Diagnostic Criteria Modified

Obsessions are defined by Criteria 1 and 2:

1. Recurrent and persistent thoughts, urges, or images that are experienced at some time during the disturbance as intrusive and unwanted, and that in most individuals cause marked anxiety or distress.
2. The individual attempts to ignore or suppress such thoughts, urges, or images, or to neutralize them with some other thought or action (i.e., by performing a compulsion).

Compulsions are defined by Criteria 1 and 2:

1. Repetitive behaviors (e.g., hand washing, ordering, checking) or mental acts (e.g., praying, counting, repeating words silently) that the individual feels driven to perform in response to an obsession or according to rules that must be applied rigidly.
2. The behaviors or mental acts are aimed at preventing or reducing anxiety or distress, or preventing some dreaded event or situation; however, they are not connected in a realistic way with what they are designed to neutralize or prevent, or are clearly excessive.

A. **Signs and Symptoms:** Presence of obsessions, compulsions, or both.
B. **Duration:** The obsessions or compulsions are time-consuming (e.g., taking more than 1 hour a day).
C. **Impairment in Function:** The symptoms cause clinically significant distress or impairment in social, occupational, or other important areas of functioning.
D. **Differential Diagnosis:**
    1. The symptoms are not attributable to the physiological effects of a substance (e.g., drug use, adverse reaction of medication) or other medical condition (e.g., Sydenham's chorea, Huntington's disease).
    2. The disturbance is not better explained by other mental disorders (e.g., obsessive-compulsive personality disorder).
    3. The disturbance is not better explained by the symptoms of GAD or other OCD-related disorders, eating disorders (EDs), substance use disorders (SUDs), or behavioral addictions (e.g., gambling).

In addition to reviewing the DSM-5 diagnostic criteria for OCD, Box 2.5 summarizes the neurobiological theories of OCD.

Box 2.5 Neurobiological Theories of Obsessive-Compulsive Disorder

Neurobiological studies of OCD have found a close correlation between clinical symptoms, cognitive function, and brain function. A large number of

---

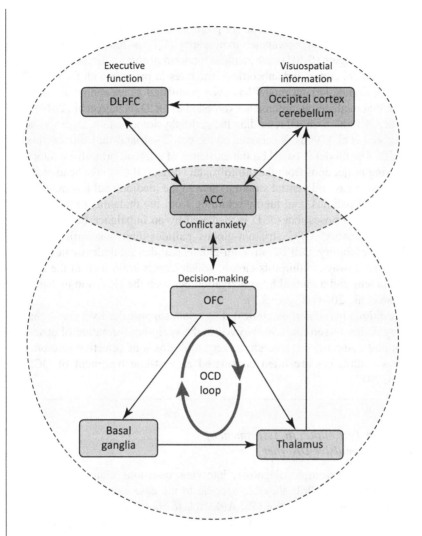

Figure 2.2 Neurobiological model of obsessive-compulsive disorder. Note: This figure describes the functional neuroanatomy of the brain in obsessive-compulsive disorder (OCD) and the correlation between brain activation and clinical improvement. A network including the dorsolateral prefrontal cortex (DLPFC), anterior cingulate cortex (ACC), and posterior regions may be related to cognitive processes in OCD, while orbitofronto-striatal regions (OCD-loop) may be involved with OCD symptomatology. Clinical improvement of OCD might accompany functional improvement of brain and cognitive improvement, such as visuospatial information, decision-making, working memory, and executive function. OFC, orbitofrontal cortex. Source: Adapted from Nakao et al. (2014).

previous neuroimaging studies using positron emission tomography (PET), single-photon emission computed tomography (CT), or functional magnetic resonance imaging (fMRI) have identified abnormally high activities throughout the frontal cortex and subcortical structures in patients with OCD. And the orbitofrontal-striatal model has been postulated as an abnormal neural circuit that mediates symptomatic expression of OCD (Nakao et al., 2014).

The OCD-loop model regarding the pathophysiology of OCD, proposed by Saxena et al. (1998), is centered on the cortico-striatal-thalamic-cortical circuits. The model is based on the existence of a lateral orbitofrontal loop involving projections from the orbitofrontal cortex (OFC) to the head of the caudate nucleus and ventral striatum, then to the mediodorsal thalamus via the internal pallidus, and finally returning from the thalamus to the OFC. The model proposes that OCD is mediated by an imbalance between the direct (excitatory, OFC striatum-globus pallidus-thalamus-cortical) and indirect (inhibitory, DLPFC-striatum-globus pallidus subthalamic nucleus-cortical) pathways within this circuit, which causes brain lock in the caudate nucleus and a mutual hyperactivation between the OFC and thalamus (Nakao et al., 2014) (Figure 2.2).

Additionally, numerous clinical drug trials support the hypothesis that dysregulation of serotonin is involved in the symptom formation of obsessions and compulsions. Therefore, very high doses of selective serotonin reuptake inhibitors are often considered as first-line treatment of OCD (Stahl, 2013).

Interviewing Techniques in Assessment of Obsessive-Compulsive Disorder

The following are sample diagnostic interview questions aimed to help elicit symptoms of OCD. While they are specific to the case exemplar that follows, they reflect the kinds of questions for APMHNs to consider during the initial psychiatric evaluation of clients, with the goal of determining whether a diagnosis of OCD based on DSM-5 symptom criteria is accurate.

The initial impression leading to the potential OCD diagnosis was based on the client's chief complaint of, "I am always worried about contracting diseases such as HIV." The APMHN noted a strong disinfectant smell from the client, which led to asking the client if he had any special cleaning linked to his concern about getting HIV. The client responded, "I have avoided touching almost anything outside of my home." This brief interaction helped the APMHN to formulate the diagnosis based on the DSM-5 symptom criteria of OCD.

- Client's chief complaint: "I am always worried about contracting diseases such as HIV." (The client had a strong disinfectant smell.)

- **APMHN:** "I noticed a smell of disinfectant; do you use any specific cleaning solution because of your concern about getting HIV?"

(The APMHN attempted to validate their own experience of disinfectant smell and to explore the client's symptom manifestations to narrow diagnosis to a specific mental disorder.)

- **Client:** "I have avoided touching almost anything outside of my home, but at times I have to use alcohol or Clorox sprays to sterilize things before and after I touch the surfaces of objects."
    (This response assists the APMHN to move toward the diagnosis of OCD, and further explore DSM-5 symptom criteria of it—presence of both obsessions and compulsions. The client met the above Definition 1 of obsession by his chief complaint of persistent worries about contracting HIV, and also met Definitions 1 and 2 of compulsion by feeling driven to avoid touching surfaces outside of the home and to use disinfectant whenever that was not possible, with the aim of preventing getting sick.)

The following are sample questions that APMHNs can incorporate into their interviews to validate information to meet the diagnostic criteria of OCD:

- Questions to validate DSM-5 diagnostic criteria of obsessions 1 and 2:
    - Would you describe in a little more detail your concerns and worries and how you manage those thoughts? For example, do you find yourself trying to ignore them or do something else to suppress them?
    - Do you ever have thoughts about specific concerns and worries that come into your mind even though you try not to think about them?
    - How hard is it to resist the thoughts or actions?
    - Do you believe these thoughts are senseless or unreasonable?
    - Do you avoid any situations that remind you of those upsetting thoughts?
- Questions to validate DSM-5 diagnostic criteria of compulsions 1 and 2:
    - Is there a time that you made a conscious effort to stop disinfecting the surface of objects before you picked them up? If you did, what happened?
    - What happens if you don't clean your hands with disinfectant after touching something?
    - Some people may pray, repeat words, or count numbers. Do you do anything like that?
    - Do you have any other ways of neutralizing the upsetting thoughts?
    - How do your compulsive actions affect your work and social/personal life?

The following is a sample case exemplar of the initial psychiatric evaluation, including how the diagnosis of OCD is determined, and the proposed treatment plan and rationales.

Case Exemplar

The client's initials are Mr. A.

A. *Identification, Chief Complaint, and Reason for Referral*

Mr. A, a 22-year-old male, came to the mental health clinic for treatment of anxiety. He was self-referred, stating that his anxiety over contracting a disease like HIV had become overwhelming and out of control, affecting his work and social life.

B. *History of the Present Illness*

At the beginning of the interview, the APMHN notes a strong disinfectant odor, and asks Mr. A if he used any cleaning disinfectant because of his concern about getting HIV. Mr. A states that all his life he has had fears and anxieties over catching germs, and he remembered washing his hands frequently, but they did not affect his daily functions and social life, as he was able to work and to have a relationship. He works full-time as a janitor, and he is glad that his job requires him to wear gloves and a mask. However, he is engaged in very few activities outside of work. Although he enjoys the company of others, he spends most of his free time at home out of fear that if he was invited out to a meal or to another person's home, the thought of touching something would be too much for him to handle. He knows that his fears and urges are "crazy and not normal." His symptoms got worse a year ago after one of his close friends died from HIV. He reported that he avoids touching almost anything outside of his home; if he even comes close to things that he thinks might have been in contact with germs, he washes his hands many times with bleach. He often washes his hands up to 30 times a day, spending hours on this routine. He tries to avoid all direct physical contact during grocery shopping, and taking the subway to work has been a big problem, due to fear and anxiety over catching germs from other people. For the last several months, he has given up attending all social events and recently his long-time girlfriend threatened to leave him unless he got some help, so he decided to seek help today.

C. *Psychiatric History/Treatment/Hospitalizations*

No past history of psychiatric treatment reported, either outpatient or inpatient in a hospital setting.

D. *Substance Use History*

Denied illicit drug use, including tobacco, denied drinking alcohol.

E. *Social and Developmental History*

1. *Education*: High school drop-out in ninth grade.
2. *Family Relationship, Social Network, and Abuse History*: Born in New York City and is an only child. Both parents are alive, but he has no close contact with them. Mr. A lives alone in a studio apartment and has a steady girlfriend. Highly limited social life due to his fear and anxiety. Denied a history of physical or sexual abuse.

3. *Legal Records*: No history of arrest or any pending legal case.
4. *Religious Background*: Christian.

F. **Family History**

No history of psychiatric illness among family and relatives reported. But Mr. A recalled that his father was always cleaning around the house and washing his hands excessively while he was growing up.

G. **Review of Systems**

1. Vital signs: BP: 120/80; HR: 70; RR: 20; Temp: 98 F; Ht: 5'8"; Wt: 150 lbs.
2. Review of systems showed no significant observable overall physical abnormalities except skin on both hands is dry, chapped, and raw from frequent washing with bleach.
3. Allergies: No known allergies reported.
4. Had a physical examination by the primary care provider a week ago and reported to be "healthy" (will obtain the copy of the physical examination).

H. **Mental Status Examination**

1. *Appearance and Behavior*: The client was a neatly dressed, 22-year-old Caucasian male, who appeared to be the stated age. He was cooperative and made good eye contact with the interviewer throughout the entire interview.
2. *Mood*: Anxious.
3. *Affect*: Irritable, mildly tense, and mood congruent.
4. *Thought Content and Process*: Speech was fluent with normal tone and volume, linear and goal directed, and coherent. Thought contents indicated no evidence of loose associations, tangential thought, thought blocking, or other signs of formal thought disorders, including delusions or ideas of reference. Denied suicidal or homicidal ideations/intents/ plans. However, recurrent and persistent thoughts of contracting HIV, followed by compulsive hand washing, are evident.
5. *Perceptual Disturbances*: Denied any form of perceptual disturbances, including auditory, visual, or tactile hallucinations.
6. *Sensorium, Cognitive, and Intellectual Functioning*: Alert and oriented × 3. There was no evidence of gross cognitive dysfunction at any point during the interview. The client acknowledged that he is often distracted from his work due to fear and anxiety over contamination, which leads to excessive hand washing.

I. **DSM-5 Diagnosis and Treatment Plan**

1. **DSM-5 Diagnosis**: Obsessive-compulsive disorder.
2. **Rationale for Diagnostic Impression**: According to the DSM-5 (APA, 2013), the following criteria must be present in order to diagnose OCD. Mr. A meets those criteria, as indicated by the bold symptom categories A–D:
   A. **Presence of obsessions and compulsions**. Mr. A has obsession manifested by the persistent thoughts of contamination, with fear of contracting HIV (definition of obsession 1). This causes Mr. A to avoid

leaving his apartment or engaging in social relationships (definition of obsession 2). He also has compulsion: repetitive and excessive hand washing (definition of compulsion 1), and the presence of anxiety and distress prior to hand washing (definition of compulsion 2).

B. ***Time-consuming.*** Washing his hands up to 30 times a day, spending hours on this as a daily routine.

C. ***Impairment in function.*** His obsessive and compulsive behaviors have led to social isolation, a strain on his relationship with his girlfriend, and are a health hazard, as demonstrated by a skin condition on both hands.

D. ***Differential diagnosis.*** Mr. A reported no known substance abuse, medical condition, or other mental disorders that may contribute to OCD symptoms.

In conclusion, the APMHN concluded that Mr. A met the DSM-5 diagnostic Criteria A, B, C, and D of obsessive-compulsive disorder.

3. ***Treatment Plan:*** OCD is a disabling psychopathology and there are different ways to treat it, primarily through:

- Psychotherapies (e.g., cognitive behavioral therapy, exposure and response prevention [ERP] therapy, and brief strategic therapy).
- Psychopharmacology (antidepressants).

(Adapted from Pietrabissa et al., 2016).

Section 6: Trauma- and Stressor-Related Disorders

The DSM-5 groups together "trauma- and stressor-related disorders" as a category for individuals who have been exposed to a traumatic and/or stressful event, and who exhibit the most prominent clinical characteristics of internalizing anhedonic and dysphoric symptoms and/or externalizing angry and aggressive symptoms, or who exhibit dissociative symptoms. Five disorders are included under this category: (1) reactive attachment disorder; (2) disinhibited social engagement disorder; (3) post-traumatic stress disorder (PTSD); (4) acute stress disorder (ASD); and (5) adjustment disorder (APA, 2013). Due to the complex developmental circumstances of childhood, the DSM-5 indicates that the diagnosis of reactive attachment disorder should be made with caution in children older than 5 years; it further reports that disinhibited social engagement disorder has not been described in adults. Therefore, these two diagnoses are excluded here, as this book solely targets adult populations. Please refer to the DSM-5 for detailed information about them.

The lifetime prevalence of PTSD is estimated to be 8% in the general population: 10% in women and 4% in men. ASD tends to be identified in less than 20% of cases following traumatic events. Its prevalence following interpersonal traumatic events, such as rape, assault, and/or witnessing a mass shooting, is 20–50%, and following non-interpersonal traumatic events is as follows: motor vehicle accidents (13–21%), mild traumatic brain injury (14%), severe burns (10%), and industrial accidents (6–12%). The prevalence of adjustment disorders varies widely from approximately 5% to 20%, depending on the population studied and the assessment methods used (APA, 2013).

Both PTSD and ASD are marked by increased stress and anxiety following direct or indirect exposure to a traumatic or stressful event (e.g., violent accident, crime, military combat, or assault, being kidnapped, being involved in a natural disaster, or experiencing systematic physical or sexual abuse). The individual reacts to the experience with fear and helplessness, persistently relives the event (e.g., in dreams and/or flashbacks), and tries to avoid being reminded of it. For ASD, the symptom pattern occurs within 3 days to 1 month after experiencing the event and resolves within that 1-month period, while for PTSD, the symptom pattern usually occurs within 3 months after experiencing the event and persists for more than 1 month (APA, 2013). Adjustment disorders are characterized by an emotional response to a stressful event, followed by symptom development. The common stressors for adult links to adjustment disorders involve financial issues, a medical illness, or a relational problem (Sadock et al., 2019). Although there are different diagnostic criteria for different trauma- and stressor-related disorders, all of these disorders have overlapping symptoms of anxiety and fear, coupled with different etiology. Table 2.14 summarizes the differential diagnosis among trauma- and stressor-related disorders.

In this section, PTSD is selected due to its association with high levels of social, occupational, and physical disability, as well as its considerable economic costs and high levels of medical utilization (APA, 2016).

Table 2.14 Differential Diagnosis among Trauma- and Stressor-Related Disorders

Diagnosis	Onset of Symptoms Following Trauma or Stressor	Duration of Symptom Manifestation	Common Trauma or Stressor
PTSD	Begins usually within the first 3 months	Varies from 3 months to more than 50 years	Violent accident, crime, military combat, assault, kidnapping, natural disaster, systematic physical or sexual abuse, motor vehicle accidents, rape, industrial accidents
ASD	Begins within 3 days to 1 month. However, ASD can't be diagnosed until 3 days after trauma	Symptoms resolve within a 1-month period	
Adjustment disorder	Begins within 3 months	Symptoms last no longer than 6 months after the stressor has ceased; if the stressor persists, symptoms become persistent	Financial issues, medical illness, relational problems

Diagnostic Criteria

DSM-5 PTSD Diagnostic Criteria Modified

A. **Etiology:** Exposure to actual or threatened death, serious injury, or sexual violence in one (or more) of the following ways:
   1. Directly experiencing the traumatic event(s).
   2. Witnessing, in person, the event(s) as it/they occurred to others.
   3. Learning that the traumatic event(s) occurred to a close family member or friend; the event(s) must have been violent or accidental.
   4. Experiencing repeated or extreme exposure to aversive details of the traumatic event(s).
B. **Signs and Symptoms:** Four major domains of symptom criteria are (1) intrusion, (2) avoidance, (3) negative alterations in cognition and mood, and (4) alterations in arousal and reactivity.
   B1. Presence of one (or more) of the following intrusion symptoms associated with the traumatic event(s), beginning after the traumatic event(s) occurred:
      1. Recurrent, involuntary, and intrusive distressing memories of the traumatic event(s).
      2. Recurrent distressing dreams in which the content and/or affect of the dream are related to the traumatic event(s).
      3. Dissociative reactions (e.g., flashbacks) in which the individual feels or acts as if the traumatic event(s) were recurring. (Such reactions may occur on a continuum, with the most extreme expression being a complete loss of awareness of present surroundings.)
      4. Intense or prolonged psychological distress at exposure to internal or external cues that symbolize or resemble an aspect of the traumatic event(s).
      5. Marked physiological reactions to internal or external cues that symbolize or resemble an aspect of the traumatic event(s).
   B2. Persistent avoidance of stimuli associated with the traumatic event(s), beginning after the traumatic event(s) occurred, as evidenced by one or both of the following:
      1. Avoidance of or efforts to avoid distressing memories, thoughts, or feelings about or closely associated with the traumatic event(s).
      2. Avoidance of or efforts to avoid external reminders (people, places, conversations, activities, objects, situations) that arouse distressing memories, thoughts, or feelings about or closely associated with the traumatic event(s).
   B3. Negative alterations in cognitions and mood associated with the traumatic event(s), beginning or worsening after the traumatic event(s) occurred, as evidenced by two (or more) of the following:

1. Inability to remember an important aspect of the traumatic event(s), typically due to dissociative amnesia, but not to other factors, such as head injury, alcohol, or drugs.
2. Persistent and exaggerated negative beliefs or expectations about oneself, others, or the world (e.g., "I am bad," "No one can be trusted," "The world is completely dangerous," "My whole nervous system is permanently ruined").
3. Persistently distorted cognitions about the cause or consequences of the traumatic events(s) that lead the individual to blame themselves or others.
4. Persistent negative emotional state (e.g., fear, horror, anger, guilt, or shame).
5. Markedly diminished interest or participation in significant activities.
6. Feelings of detachment or estrangement from others.
7. Persistent inability to experience positive emotions (e.g., inability to experience happiness, satisfaction, or loving feelings).

B4. Marked alterations in arousal and reactivity associated with the traumatic event(s), beginning or worsening after the traumatic event(s) occurred, as evidenced by two (or more) of the following:

1. Irritable behavior and angry outbursts with little or no provocation, typically expressed as verbal or physical aggression toward people or objects.
2. Reckless or self-destructive behavior.
3. Hypervigilance.
4. Exaggerated startle response.
5. Problems with concentration.
6. Sleep disturbance.

C. **Duration:** PTSD signs and symptoms are present for more than 1 month.
D. **Impairment in Function:** The signs and symptoms cause clinically significant distress or impairment in social, occupational, or other important areas of functioning.
E. **Differential Diagnosis:** The symptoms are not attributable to the physiological effects of a substance (e.g., drug use, adverse reaction of medication) or other medical condition.

In addition to the review of the differential diagnosis among trauma- and stressor-related disorders, it is essential that APMHNs have a working knowledge of its neurobiological basis, especially the role of brain circuits and related symptom dimensions, in order to understand how psychotropic medications have been used in its treatment. Box 2.6 briefly summarizes the neurobiological aspect of PTSD.

Box 2.6 Neurobiological Theories of Post-Traumatic Stress Disorder

Although there are different diagnostic criteria for different trauma- and stressor-related disorders, all of these disorders have overlapping symptoms of anxiety and fear, coupled with different etiology. Trauma- and stressor-related symptoms are regulated by an amygdala-centered circuit; circuit malfunctioning may be traumatic in origin and conditioned in post-traumatic stress disorder (Stahl, 2013). The core characteristic symptoms of PTSD are anxiety while the traumatic event is being re-experienced, increased arousal, startle responses, sleep difficulties, including nightmares, and avoidance behaviors. Table 2.15 presents the core symptoms of PTSD in relation to the effected brain regions and circuits.

Table 2.15 Symptoms of PTSD in Brain Regions and Circuits

Core symptoms of PTSD	*Overactivation of* **amygdala** *circuit reciprocal or activating connection with*
Traumatic re-experiencing	• Traumatic memories stored in the hippocampus can activate the amygdala, causing the amygdala, in turn, to activate other brain regions and generate a fear response
Avoidance behaviors	• Avoidance is a motor response which is regulated by reciprocal connections between the amygdala and periaqueductal gray
Increased arousal	• Dysfunctional hypothalamic–pituitary–adrenal (HPA) axis
Startle responses; fight/flight or freeze	• Malfunctioning parabrachial nucleus (PBN) plays a major role in transmitting real or potential threat signals to the extended amygdala
Linking "fear" to amygdala circuits to neurotransmitters and voltage-gated iron channels	• Malfunctioning of amygdala-centered circuits, which are regulated by neurotransmitters (serotonin, GABA, glutamate, norepinephrine) and voltage-gated iron channels
Sleep difficulties, including nightmares	• Dysfunctional HPA axis and anatomical alterations in the hippocampus

Source: Adapted from Stahl (2013).

Interviewing Techniques in Assessment of Post-Traumatic Stress Disorder

The following are examples of diagnostic interview questions for APMHNs to consider during the initial psychiatric evaluation of a client to help elicit the symptoms of PTSD and to formulate the final diagnosis based on a full mental health assessment. The sample questions are based on the etiology of the trauma, such as a complicated childbirth, and the resulting symptoms that affect social and familial lives.

Question #1: I see that it's hard for you to talk about what happened during the delivery of your baby. Of course, I can review your medical records, but I would like to hear from you the way you experienced it. If not right now, maybe later. For now, would you share how the event has been affecting your life for the last 6 months?

(Initially, building a rapport with the client while understanding and accepting her hesitance to share, but at the same time guiding the client to the importance of sharing her problems when she is ready. Meanwhile, tap on the post-traumatic experience with an open-ended question.)

Question #2: Do you ever experience an overwhelming feeling related to the event forcing its way into your mind?

Question #3: Do you ever have nightmares about the event?

Question #4: Do you ever experience flashbacks, like reliving visual or emotional memories of the event?

Question #5: Do you ever feel like it's happening all over again?

(Questions 2–5 are questions to explore intrusive symptoms associated with the trauma.)

Question #6: Do you find yourself avoiding things that remind you of the event?

Question #7: How hard is it for you to talk about the event?

Question #8: Have you been avoiding activities that you used to enjoy?

(Questions 6–8 are questions to explore avoidance symptoms associated with the trauma.)

Question #9: Would you share how the event has been affecting your life?

Question #10: Have your friendships suffered?

Question #11: Are you still able to feel the same way toward your loved ones as before?

Question #12: Have you ever experienced numbness since the event?

Question #13: Do you enjoy things that you used to enjoy since the event?

(Questions 9–13 are questions to explore alterations in cognitions and mood associated with the trauma.)

Question #14: Do you feel on edge more often than not since the event?

Question #15: Do you find that you startle easily?

Question #16: Do you sleep well at night?

Question #17: Do you find yourself having a hard time focusing or concentrating?

(Questions 14–17 are questions related to alterations in arousal and reactivity associated with the trauma.)

The following is a sample case exemplar of the initial psychiatric evaluation, including how the diagnosis of PTSD is determined, with the proposed treatment plan and rationales.

Case Exemplar

The client's initials are SG.

A. *Identification, Chief Complaint, and Reason for Referral*

SG is a 22-year-old Latina female, a single mother of a 6-month-old infant. She presented to the APMHN with a complaint of low libido affecting her relationship with her boyfriend, who is the father of the baby. SG claimed that she did not want to have intercourse due to a pronounced fear related to her traumatic childbirth experience, and her primary care provider referred her to the mental health clinic for psychiatric evaluation.

B. *History of the Present Illness*

SG was highly reluctant to discuss what happened during the delivery of her daughter 6 months ago; therefore, the APMHN obtained and reviewed the client's medical records, with her consent. According to the records, SG had an uncomplicated pregnancy, but was admitted to the hospital 1 week after her due date for an induction of labor, which took 3 days. SG went through extensive medical procedures and medications (cervidil PV, a cervical balloon, artificial rupture of membranes, and pitocin IV) without relief of pain. Additionally, she developed preeclampsia with a severe range of blood pressures, requiring emergency intervention with medications (magnesium sulfate and labetalol). On day three, she reached full dilatation and pushed for 2 hours, at which time a prolonged fetal heart rate deceleration was noted and an emergency cesarean section was performed. The neonate was sent to the neonatal intensive care unit (NICU) and remained there for 3 days for meconium aspiration syndrome. SG also had a postpartum hemorrhage in the operating room (OR) and required a transfusion of 2 L packed red blood cells.

Since the birth of her child, SG reported difficulty sleeping and frequent nightmares re-experiencing her hospital experience. She has been on edge all the time and easily startled. Memories of the baby's birth are often so intrusive that they literally take over her life when they come, "like nightmares, but I'm awake." She has avoided not only the hospital where she had the baby, but all hospitals, walking far out of her way to not see them. She won't go to her daughter's pediatrician appointments due to the anticipation that that would provoke memories of the baby's birth (SG's mother takes her to the appointments). Additionally, SG has avoided two of her close friends who were pregnant, saying "seeing them brings me too many memories."

She feels disconnected from her friends and thinks they wouldn't understand what she has been through and would think she was weak and should have done things differently. SG's mother has been staying with her to take care of the baby, and reported that SG is overprotective of her daughter, as she rarely lets the baby out of her sight. "Everything I do is to keep her safe." At the same time, she does not feel joy or love for her daughter. Rather, she only experiences fear and anxiety, which leads to the overly protective behaviors. Initially, SG admitted that she did not feel connected to her daughter and in the first few days of her life she rarely saw her, which she feels guilty about. SG has been feeling "distant" from her boyfriend in addition to avoiding physical intimacy. Her boyfriend complained to her that since the birth of their daughter she won't talk to him anymore and only snaps at him. She agreed with the boyfriend's comments, saying that she often doesn't even hear what he is saying because she is spaced out and then he gets annoyed with her.

She has been angry and does not trust the medical system, saying, "I was so stupid before. I just trusted everyone to take care of me and my baby, but it doesn't work like that." She admitted that she has not been herself since the birth of her daughter, and has been feeling "on edge" all the time and is easily startled.

SG denied suicidal ideation/intent/plan and reported no delusions or hallucinations. She recognizes that she cannot continue to live as she currently is. She would like to be able to stop having flashbacks and intrusive memories and wants to have a "normal" relationship with her boyfriend and be able to relax and enjoy being a mother. She misses her friends and wants to feel at ease around them again.

C. *Psychiatric History/Rx/Hospitalizations*

No past history of psychiatric treatments was reported, either outpatient or in an inpatient hospital setting. No prior diagnosed psychiatric symptoms before the onset of the current episode.

D. *Substance Use History*

SG denies tobacco or illicit drug use, and used to have two to three drinks socially at parties.

E. *Social and Developmental History*

1. *Education:* Completion of graduate program in education.
2. *Family Relationship, Social Network, and Abuse History*: SG is an only child and her parents divorced when she was 10 years old. Following the divorce, she lived with her mother. SG claimed that she was sexually assaulted by her mother's boyfriend when she was 15 years old and she went to live with her father. However, she did not disclose the incident until she was 17, after her mother had broken up with the perpetrator. They never pressed charges as "he had moved back to his country." She did not seek any help at the time since her mother and her friends helped her get through the trauma. Currently, she is living with her boyfriend who has been supportive of her, and the mother has been helping her to take care of the newborn baby.
3. *Legal Records*: No history of arrest or any pending legal case.
4. *Religious Background*: Christian.

F. *Family History*

SG denies any family history of mental illness or medical issues.

G. *Review of Systems*

1. Vital signs: BP: 110/60; HR: 80; RR: 24; Temp: 98 F; Ht: 5'5"; Wt: 125 lbs.
2. Review of systems showed no significant observable overall physical abnormalities.
3. Allergies: No known allergies reported.
4. Monthly visits to OB/GYN for close monitoring of anemia due to hemorrhage during childbirth and postpartum care. The last visit was a week ago and SG reported that she was informed that she has made a full physical recovery, but was recommended to seek mental health care.

H. *Mental Status Examination*

1. *Appearance and Behavior*: The client was a neatly dressed, 22-year-old Latina female, who appeared to be the stated age. Overall, she was cooperative during the interview but initially hesitant to engage in the conversation and avoided eye contact with the interviewer.
2. *Mood*: Anxious.
3. *Affect*: Guided and mood congruent.
4. *Thought Content and Process*: Speech was fluent with normal tone of voice, and linear, goal directed, and coherent. Thought contents indicated no evidence of loose associations, tangential thought, thought blocking, or other signs of a formal thought disorder, including delusions or ideas of reference. Denied suicidal or homicidal ideations/intents/plans.
5. *Perceptual Disturbances*: Denied any forms of perceptual disturbances, including auditory, visual, or tactile hallucinations.
6. *Sensorium, Cognitive, and Intellectual Functioning*: Alert and oriented × 3. There was no evidence of gross cognitive dysfunction at any point during the interview. The client is insightful of her fear and anxiety related to what occurred during childbirth, and of its impact on her life in general.

I. *Diagnosis and Treatment Plan*

1. **DSM-5 Diagnosis:** Post-traumatic stress disorder.
2. **Rationale for Diagnostic Impression:** According to the DSM-5 (APA, 2013), the following criteria must be present to diagnose PTSD. SG meets these criteria, as indicated by the bold symptom categories A–F:
    A. **Etiology: *Directly experiencing the traumatic events.*** This criterion was met with the client's traumatic near-death experience from the complicated medical crises during the 3-day delivery of her baby.
    B. **Signs and Symptoms:**
    B1. **Intrusion Symptoms:** Presence of one (or more) of the following intrusion symptoms associated with the traumatic event(s), beginning after the traumatic event(s) occurred:
       1. ***Recurrent, involuntary, and intrusive distressing memories of the traumatic event(s).*** SG often experienced the intrusive distressing memories of the baby's birth.

2. *Recurrent distressing dreams* in which the content and/or effect of the dream are related to the traumatic event(s). SG reported difficulty sleeping, with frequent nightmares re-experiencing her traumatic event when she was in the hospital.

3. *Dissociative reactions* (e.g., flashbacks) in which the individual feels or acts as if the traumatic event(s) were recurring. SG often didn't even hear what her boyfriend was saying to her because she was "spaced out." And memories of the baby's birth were often so intrusive that they literally took over her life when they came, "like nightmares, but I'm awake."

4. *Intense or prolonged psychological distress* at exposure to internal or external cues that symbolize or resemble an aspect of the traumatic event(s). When SG saw two of her close friends who were pregnant, it brought back too many memories of her own childbirth experience.

5. Marked physiological reactions to internal or external cues that symbolize or resemble an aspect of the traumatic event(s).

SG's symptoms meet four out of five (requires two or more) symptom categories of B1 (1, 2, 3, 4).

B2. **Persistent Avoidance Symptoms:** Persistent avoidance of stimuli associated with the traumatic events, beginning after the traumatic event(s) occurred, as evidenced by one or both of the following:

1. *Avoidance* of or efforts to avoid distressing memories, *thoughts*, or *feelings* about or closely associated with the traumatic event(s). Socially, SG has avoided two of her close friends who were pregnant, saying "seeing them brings me too many memories."

2. *Avoidance* of or efforts to avoid *external reminders* (people, places, conversations, activities, objects, situations) that arouse distressing memories, thoughts, or feelings about or closely associated with the traumatic event(s). SG has avoided not only the hospital where she was treated but all hospitals by walking far out of her way to not see them. She won't go to her daughter's pediatrician appointments due to the anticipation that that would provoke memories of the baby's birth. SG's mother takes her daughter to the appointments.

SG's symptoms meet both (requires one or both) B2 symptom categories (1, 2).

B3. **Negative Alterations in Cognition and Mood:** Negative alterations in cognition and mood associated with the traumatic event(s), beginning or worsening after the traumatic event(s) occurred, as evidenced by two (or more) of the following:

1. *Persistent and exaggerated negative beliefs or expectations* about oneself, *others*, or the world. "I was so stupid before. I just trusted everyone to take care of me and my baby, but it doesn't work like that"; "I was weak and should have done things differently."

2. *Persistent negative emotional state* (e.g., fear, horror, anger, guilt, or shame). SG has been angry toward the medical team, and

feels guilty over her continuing lack of feelings toward the baby, and sad about not being able to enjoy her baby as she thinks she should.

3. *Markedly diminished interest or participation in significant activities.* SG is isolating herself by not going out with her friends, and by lack of interest in engaging in physical intimacy with her boyfriend.

4. *Persistent inability to experience positive emotions* (e.g., inability to experience happiness, satisfaction, or loving feelings). SG has been feeling guilty that she has no feelings of joy or love toward the baby. Her fear and anxiety have led her to be overprotective of her daughter, as she rarely lets the baby out of her sight.

SG's symptoms meet four (requires two or more) B3 symptom categories (1, 2, 3, 4).

B4. **Marked alterations in arousal and reactivity:** Associated with the traumatic event(s), beginning or worsening after the traumatic event(s) occurred, as evidenced by two (or more) of the following:

1. *Irritable behavior and angry outbursts* with little or no provocation, typically expressed as verbal or physical aggression toward people or objects. Her boyfriend complains to her that since the birth of their daughter, she won't talk to him and only snaps at him.

2. Reckless or self-destructive behavior.

3. *Hypervigilance.* She has been feeling "on edge" all the time.

4. *Exaggerated startle response.* SB has been easily startled.

5. Problems with concentration.

6. *Sleep disturbance.* SB has been experiencing difficulty sleeping, with frequent nightmares.

SG's symptoms meet four (requires two or more) of the B4 symptom categories (1, 3, 4, 6).

C. **Duration:** PTSD signs and symptoms are present for *more than 1 month*. SG's PTSD symptoms have been present persistently for 6 months since the delivery of the baby.

D. **Impairment in Function:** The signs and symptoms cause clinically *significant distress or impairment* in social, occupational, or other important areas of functioning. SG has not been able to function independently due to the current symptoms, and requires assistance with childcare from her mother. Her social activities are highly affected, as she avoids seeing her friends.

E. **Differential Diagnosis:** The symptoms are not attributable to the physiological effects of a substance (e.g., drug use, medication) or medical condition. SG denied any history of substance use and no treatable medical conditions other than postpartum care.

In conclusion, the APMHN concluded that SG met the DSM-5 diagnostic criteria for PTSD.

3. ***Treatment Plan and Summary*:**

Postpartum PTSD can adversely affect women's well-being, mother–infant relationships, and child development. Treatment plans for the PTSD client in general:

- The emphasis should be on education about the disorder and treatment for it, both psychotherapeutic and psychopharmacological. At any point during assessment or treatment, pressing a client to talk about a trauma who is reluctant to do so would be counterproductive and may exacerbate symptom manifestations (Sadock et al., 2019).
- In terms of psychotherapy, trauma-focused psychological interventions (TFPT), including exposure therapy, trauma-focused cognitive behavioral therapy, and eye-movement desensitization and reprocessing (EMDR) were reported to be effective in reducing postpartum PTSD symptoms in both the short- (up to 3 months postpartum) and medium- (3–6 months postpartum) term. However, no robust evidence suggests that TFPT can also improve women's recovery from clinically significant postpartum PTSD symptoms (Furuta et al., 2018).
- Psychopharmacological interventions are also reported to be effective; the use of selective serotonin reuptake inhibitors and tricyclic agents is supported by a number of well-controlled clinical trials (Sadock et al., 2019).
- Additional support for the client and family can be obtained through local and national support groups for clients with PTSD.

Section 7: Feeding and Eating Disorders

Feeding and eating disorders are characterized by persistent disturbance of eating or eating-related behaviors that results in altered consumption or absorption of food and significantly impacts the affected individual's physical health and/or psychosocial functioning. According to the DSM-5, feeding and eating disorders include six distinctively specified disorders: (1) pica, (2) rumination disorder, (3) avoidant/restrictive food intake disorder, (4) anorexia nervosa, (5) bulimia nervosa, and (6) binge-eating disorder. Despite a number of common psychological and behavioral features, each disorder differs substantially in clinical course, outcome, and treatment needs. However, a diagnosis of pica may be assigned in the presence of any other feeding and eating disorder. Finally, obesity is not considered to be a mental disorder and therefore is not included in the DSM-5. The prevalence of pica, rumination disorder, and avoidant/restrictive food intake disorders is reported as inconclusive compared to other eating disorders. Twelve-month prevalence of anorexia nervosa among young females is approximately 0.4%, but far less common in males than in females, with an approximately 10:1 female-to-male ratio. Twelve-month prevalence of bulimia nervosa among young females is 1–1.5%, also less common in males than in females, with the same approximately 10:1 female-to-male ratio. Twelve-month prevalence of binge-eating disorder among female and male adults (age 18 or older) is 1.6% and 0.8%, respectively (APA, 2013) (Tables 2.16 and 2.17).

Table 2.16 Differential Diagnosis among Feeding and Eating Disorders

Diagnosis	Eating Pattern or Eating-Related Behavior	Diagnostic Markers
Pica	- Persistent eating of nonnutritive, nonfood substances	• Childhood onset is most commonly reported • Abdominal obstruction • Lab test to ascertain levels of poisoning or the nature of infection
Rumination disorder	- Repeated regurgitation of food - Regurgitated food may be re-chewed, re-swallowed, or spit out	• Malnutrition • Growth delay • Weight loss or low weight • Symptoms may occur in the context of intellectual disability
Avoidant/ restrictive food intake disorder	- Apparent lack of interest in eating or food - Avoidance based on sensory characteristics of food - Concern about aversive consequences of eating	• Malnutrition • Low weight • Growth delay • Need for artificial nutrition
Anorexia nervosa (AN)	- Restriction of energy intake relative to requirements by semi-starvation, purging behaviors, laxative and/or diuretic abuse, excessive physical activity	• Leukopenia, mild anemia • Hypercholesterolemia • Elevated hepatic enzyme • Metabolic alkalosis • Metabolic acidosis • Low serum mineral level (magnesium, zinc, phosphate) • Elevated amylase level
Bulimia nervosa (BN)	- Recurrent episodes of binge eating in a discrete period of time - Recurrent inappropriate compensatory behaviors in order to prevent weight gain—e.g., self-induced vomiting, misuse of laxatives, diuretics, fasting, excessive exercise	• Electrolyte abnormalities • Metabolic alkalosis • Metabolic acidosis • Permanent loss of dental enamel • Cardiac and skeletal myopathies
Binge-eating disorder (BED)	- Recurrent episodes of binge eating and lack of control over eating during the episode - Not associated with inappropriate compensatory behaviors	• Weight gain • Crossover from binge-eating disorder to other eating disorders is uncommon • Dysfunctional dieting usually precedes the onset of binge eating

Source: Adapted from DSM-5, APA (2013).

Table 2.17 Indications of High Medical Risk and Inpatient Treatment

Indication	Medical Risk
Weight	BMI <14 kg/m² or rapid weight loss
Medical status	Heart rate <50 bpm, cardiac arrhythmia, postural tachycardia (increase >20 bpm), blood pressure <80/50 mm Hg, postural hypotension >20 mm Hg, QTc >450 ms, temperature <35.5°C, hypokalemia <3.0 mmol/L, neutropenia, phosphate <0.5 mmol/L
Additional indicators	• Severe binge eating and purging several times daily • Failure to respond to outpatient or day-patient treatment • Severe psychiatric comorbidity • Suicidality

Source: Adapted from Hay et al. (2014).

In addition to the review of the differential diagnosis among feeding and eating disorders, it is essential that APMHNs have a working knowledge of its neurobiological basis, especially the role of the brain structure and reward pathways circuits, and altered brain activity across eating disorders. Box 2.7 presents a summary of neurobiological findings on eating disorders.

Box 2.7 Neurobiological Findings on Eating Disorders

Research on eating disorders has identified the importance of the short-term impact of ED behaviors on the brain structure, as brain reward pathways are most consistently implicated in altered brain activity across EDs (Table 2.18).

Table 2.18 Summary of Neurobiological Findings in Eating Disorders

Brain structure and reward pathways	Altered brain activity across eating disorders
Neurochemistry	• Serotonin 1A receptor increased in ill AN and BN • Serotonin 2A receptor normal in ill AN, decreased in recurrent AN • Hormones, neuropeptides altered in all EDs, often normalize with recovery; may interfere with appetite regulation and reward system • Cytokines increased in ill AN and BN; normalize with recovery
Gray matter (GM) volume and cortical thickness	• Cortical volume and thickness vary among studies in EDs, probably due to confounding factors, such as malnutrition, dehydration, comorbidity, and medication use • Lower volume or thickness in AN frequently normalize with weight restoration

White matter (WM) volume, integrity, and structural connectivity	• WM volume varies similarly to GM studies • Fractional anisotropy (FA) thought to reflect fiber integrity, tends to be lower in AN and BN • Lower FA may be compensated for in AN and BN with increased fiber development between insula and orbitofrontal cortex
Functional and effective connectivity	• Increased and decreased functional connectivity in default mode network (interoception), salience network (orientation to food stimuli), and executive control network (decision-making) in AN and BN • Effective connectivity to the hypothalamus in AN, BN may override hunger signals
Task-based fMRI studies	• Reward circuits are consistently altered to food stimuli in insula, striatum, orbitofrontal cortex • Altered prediction error response to food and monetary stimuli suggest altered dopamine circuit response in AN, BN, and BED • Perception, increased and decreased in insula, parietal, and visual cortex to interoception or visual perception tasks • AN is associated with reduced insula neural taste discrimination • Cognition tasks often increased and decreased brain response in AN although behavior response mostly normal • BN had increased striatal and worse behavior response when distracted by food images • Social interaction, gentle touch, and visual intimate stimuli were associated with decreased brain response and decreased pleasantness ratings
Microbiota and microbiome	• Decreased diversity of gut microbial cells (microbiota) in AN, may normalize with weight restoration

Source: Adapted from Frank et al. (2019).

In this section, anorexia nervosa is chosen as an example to address the mental status assessment and diagnostic evaluation of feeding and eating disorders, as it represents the classic condition in this group of disorders.

Diagnostic Criteria

DSM-5 Anorexia Nervosa Diagnostic Criteria Modified

A. **Signs and Symptoms:**

1. Restriction of energy intake relative to requirements, leading to a significantly low body weight in the context of age, sex, developmental trajectory, and physical health. Significantly low body weight is defined as weight that is less than minimally normal.
2. Intense fear of gaining weight or of becoming fat, and/or persistent behavior that interferes with weight gain, even though at a significantly low body weight.

3. Disturbance in the way in which one's body weight or shape is experienced, undue influence of body weight or shape on self-evaluation, or persistent lack of recognition of the seriousness of the current low body weight.

B. **Subtype Specifier:**

1. **Restricting type:** During the last 3 months, the individual has not engaged in recurrent episodes of binge eating or purging behaviors (e.g., self-induced vomiting or the misuse of laxatives, diuretics, or enemas). This subtype describes presentations in which weight loss is accomplished primarily through dieting, fasting, and/or excessive exercise.
2. **Binge-eating/purging type:** During the last 3 months, the individual has engaged in recurrent episodes of binge eating or purging behaviors.

C. **Remission Specifier:**

1. **In partial remission:** After full criteria for anorexia nervosa were previously met, Criterion A1 (low body weight) has not been met for a sustained period, but either Criterion A2 (intense fear of gaining weight or of becoming fat and/or behavior that interferes with weight gain) or Criterion A3 (disturbance in self-perception of body weight and shape) is still met.
2. **In full remission:** After full criteria for anorexia nervosa were previously met, none of the criteria have been met for a sustained period of time.

D. **Current Severity Specifier:**

The minimum level of severity for adults is based on current body mass index: Mild (≥ 17.0 kg/m^2 BMI), moderate (16–16.99 kg/m^2 BMI), severe (15–15.99 kg/m^2 BMI), and extreme (<15 kg/m^2 BMI). A normal body mass index is 18.5–24.9 kg/m^2.

The nutritional compromise associated with anorexia nervosa could result in physiological disturbances, such as amenorrhea and abnormal vital signs. While most of these are reversible with nutritional rehabilitation, other conditions, such as loss of bone mineral density, are often not completely reversible.

Interviewing Techniques in Assessment of Anorexia Nervosa

Clients with anorexia nervosa are usually guarded and tend to minimize their symptoms; therefore, establishing rapport is crucial at the beginning of the interview, while maintaining a high index of suspicion. If the client has difficulty responding, the APMHN needs to be more active, while being patient with this difficulty. The following questions are examples for the APMHN to consider when evaluating a client's presenting symptoms to formulate a final diagnosis of anorexia nervosa, based on the DSM-5 symptom criteria.

Criterion A1: Self-induced weight loss

Questions:

- *Sometimes people may use different ways of losing weight, such as exercise, fat burners, laxatives. How do you lose weight or prevent yourself from putting on weight? (This question is a normalizing statement to assist with information gathering.)*

Criterion A2: Morbid fear of fatness

Questions:

- *What is your height and your weight? (Calculate BMI)*
- *Are you concerned about your weight?*
- *Are you afraid of gaining weight?*
- *What have you done to prevent yourself from gaining weight?*

Criterion A3: Body image disturbance

Questions:

- *What do you think your ideal weight is?*
- *What do you see when you look in the mirror?*
- *Can you envision yourself and draw what you look like now, and what you would like to look like?*

Criterion B: Subtype specifier

Restricting type: *During the last 3 months, have you kept dieting, fasting, and/or exercising to lose weight without binge eating or purging, like forcing yourself to throw up or excessively using enemas, laxatives, or diuretics?*

Binge-eating/purging type: *During the last 3 months, have you been repeatedly binge eating or purging, like forcing yourself to throw up or excessively using enemas, laxatives, or diuretics?*

The following is a case exemplar of the initial psychiatric evaluation, including how the diagnosis of anorexia nervosa is determined, the proposed treatment plan, and rationales.

Case Exemplar

The client's initial is S.

A. ***Identification, Chief Complaint, and Reason for Referral***

S is a 25-year-old Caucasian female, employed, lives with her husband. She was brought in by her husband when she complained of fatigue, palpitations, and abdominal pain. He reported that his wife has been using laxatives regularly after she complained of constipation about 3 months ago.

B. *History of Present Illness*

S presented to a local community tertiary care center with complaints of excessive tiredness and two episodes of syncope in the last 2 months. S was hesitant to engage in the interview initially and her husband started to talk in her place. The APMHN redirected to the client with gentle probing, and she started to report her gradual loss of weight, recurrent episodes of vomiting for a period of 2 years, menstrual irregularities for 1 year, and amenorrhea for the last 6 months. According to the husband, the probable precipitating factor was when he made a critical comment about S' weight 3 years ago, during their early days of marriage. The husband claimed that he had casually made a remark about her being slightly heavy near her trunk and thighs, and that she would look more beautiful if she reduced it. Since then, her intake of food has decreased. She eventually developed a morbid fear of looking fat and ugly, and began eating a handful of fennel seeds to facilitate digestion. She would use a soap water enema and occasionally use laxatives. Her weight dropped steadily from 130 lbs to 88 lbs over the 3-year period. She completely avoided all foods with a high caloric value. She gradually began to skip breakfast and would have minimal lunch. She began to avoid eating in front of other family members. At times, she would hide and eat, and/or would secretly go into the bathroom and induce vomiting. She expressed that her mood has been down, and that she is tired, apathetic, has decreased attention and concentration, and feels empty and pessimistic about her future. S' husband concurred with what the client reported and reiterated that the client has been dull and inactive most of the time and their marriage has been in turmoil, as she has not been able to carry out her daily living adequately. With symptoms of weight loss and amenorrhea, she reported that she had a series of medical workups a month ago and that all tests were within normal limits except low hemoglobin. Based on her past history, the APMHN suspected that S might minimize her eating disorder's impact on her overall health.

C. *Past Psychiatric History*

Patient denies any history of psychiatric diagnosis and her husband also said he does not know of any mental illness. No suicidal ideas or unusual perceptual experiences were reported. However, the client was hospitalized three times for electrolyte imbalance and she was reluctant to elaborate about the reasons for the past hospitalizations.

D. *Substance Use History*

S denies any use of nicotine, alcohol, cannabis, cocaine, heroin, opiates, or benzodiazepines.

E. *Social and Developmental History*

S has been married for 3 years and is living with her husband, who works as an accountant in the local bank. She completed her master's degree from Baruch College and currently works as an accountant at Chase Bank. S was always a high achiever academically; she graduated at the top of her class in college, and performed academically excellently in high school and elementary school. She is the youngest child of two children and reported no developmental issues. Her family is Anglican and she meditates religiously every Sunday.

F. *Family Relationships, Social Network, and Abuse History*

S's parents have been married for 28 years and own a boating business in New Rochelle. The client claimed that she has a close relationship with her parents and sister, and remembers her childhood with fond memories of rock climbing and family vacations. She denies any kind of domestic violence, or past history of abuse or maltreatment.

G. *Work/Legal/Military History*

S works as an accountant at the local Chase Bank. She denies any legal history or any pending legal problem, and has no military record.

H. *Family Psychiatric History*

S reports a history of depression in the family. Her mother's brother was diagnosed and treated for depression between 2012 and 2015. Her father's brother has a history of polysubstance use disorder and was admitted to the hospital for treatment several times without success; he died of a heroin overdose in 2018.

I. *Medical History and Review of Systems*

1. Vital signs: BP: 90/50; HR: 60; RR: 18; Temp: 97 F; Ht: 5'4"; Wt: 88 lbs; BMI 15.6 kg/m^2.
2. General: Alert, awake, and oriented × 4 to name, place, time, purpose; thin body frame, poorly nourished.
3. Hair and nail: Brittle.
4. Allergies: No known allergies reported.
5. During the interview, S was recommended hospitalization for a thorough physical examination and treatment of her eating disorder. However, she declined the recommendation and also refused to have a physical examination following the interview, other than taking vital signs. Instead, she agreed to see her PCP for a full physical examination and consented for the APMHN to contact her PCP to obtain a copy of her medical records.

J. *Mental Status Examination*

1. *Appearance and Behavior*: S appeared to be her age, with an extremely thin body frame. She had lanugo hair on her face, which is common for a person with an eating disorder. Her hygiene was clean, but she was overly dressed, wearing four layers of clothing and a big sweater, as she claimed that she is cold all the time. During the interview, her overall attitude and behavior appeared to be uncomfortable and resistant, and her presentation was unpleasant and guarded. However, as the interview progressed, she became cooperative and engaged marginally in the conversation.
2. *Mood*: Depressed and anxious.
3. *Affect*: Irritable, easily fatigued, and apathetic.

4. *Thought Content and Process*: Speech was fluent and articulate, volume was soft and monotonous. No thought blocking was noted, and overall thought process was linear and logical.
5. *Perceptual Disturbances*: S denied delusions or hallucinations, and denied homicidal/suicidal ideations, intention, or plans.
6. *Sensorium, Cognitive, and Intellectual Functioning*: Alert and oriented × 4. Her concentration was fair and she was able to calculate serial 3s from 20 with ease. She was able to spell MEMORY backward. Recent and remote memories were intact, and she was able to recall three out of three unrelated items (apple, table, and penny) after 1 minute and after 5 minutes.

K. *Diagnosis and Treatment Plan*

1. *DSM-5 Diagnosis*: Anorexia nervosa.
2. *Rationale for Diagnostic Impression*: According to the DSM-5 (APA, 2013), the following criteria must be present to diagnose anorexia nervosa. The client met those criteria, as indicated by the bold symptom categories A–F:

A. **Signs and Symptoms:**
1. *Restriction of energy intake relative to requirements, leading to a significant low body weight* in the context of age, sex, developmental trajectory, and physical health. Significantly low weight is defined as weight that is less than minimally normal.

   The client's weight dropped from 130 lbs to 88 lbs over 3 years. She followed a change in diet pattern with complete avoidance of all foods with a high caloric value. She gradually began to skip breakfast and would have minimal lunch.
2. *Intense fear of gaining weight or of becoming fat, and/or persistent behavior that interferes with weight gain*, even though at a significantly low weight.

   The client eventually developed a morbid fear of looking fat and ugly, would use soap water enemas, and would occasionally use laxatives.
3. Disturbance in the way in which one's body weight or shape is experienced, undue influence of body weight or shape on self-evaluation, or **persistent lack of recognition of the seriousness of the current low body weight**.

   The client was hospitalized three times for electrolyte imbalance, but was reluctant to elaborate on the reasons for the past hospitalizations.

B. **Subtype Specifier:**
   Binge-eating/purging type: During the last 3 months, the individual has engaged in recurrent episodes of binge eating or purging behaviors.

   At times, the client would hide and eat, and/or would secretly go into the bathroom and induce vomiting.

C. **Current Severity Specifier:**
   The minimum level of severity for adults is based on current body mass index: mild (≥ 17.0 kg/m^2 BMI), moderate (16–16.99 kg/m^2 BMI), severe (15–15.99 kg/m^2 BMI), and extreme (<15 kg/m^2 BMI).

The client is 5'4" in height and weighs (fully clothed with four layers and a heavy sweater) 88 lbs. Minus the weight of the clothes (3–4 lbs), her actual weight is 84 or 85 lbs (BMI: 15.6), which indicates the current severity specifier for this client is "severe."

The APMHN concluded that the client met the DSM-5 diagnostic criteria as addressed above for anorexia nervosa, binge-eating/purging type, severe.

3. ***Treatment Plan and Summary***:

Based on the severity of the client's symptoms, the APMHN recommended that she first be admitted to an inpatient medical unit for a full diagnostic workup, including pathology and laboratory examination, to be stabilized medically first, and then referred for outpatient treatment for an eating disorder. The client declined the recommendation, but agreed to see her PCP for the workup.

Individuals with anorexia nervosa who are 20% below the expected weight for their height are recommended for inpatient programs; those who are 30% below their expected weight require psychiatric hospitalization for 2–6 months (Sadock et al., 2019). This client's expected weight for her height (5'4") is 107 lbs, but her current weight without clothes is approximately 84 lbs, which is 20% below her expected weight and warrants an inpatient program. The first consideration in the treatment of anorexia nervosa is to restore the client's nutritional state, and in her present state of mind the client cannot take care of herself, especially in terms of her needed dietary intake. A family meeting with the husband will be held to discuss the options for the client's treatment plan and to provide education related to eating disorders and their impact on overall physical and mental health, with suitable recommendations for the client's current condition.

Section 8: Substance-Related and Addictive Disorders

Substance-related and addictive disorders cause significant disabilities and affect multiple areas of functioning for a relatively high percentage of the population. Lipari and Van Horn (2017) reported that in 2014, approximately 20.2 million adults aged 18 or older had a past year substance use disorder, 16.3 million had an alcohol use disorder (AUD), and 6.2 million had an illicit drug use disorder (DUD), with an estimated 2.3 million adults having both an AUD and an illicit DUD in the previous year. A November 2015 National Institutes of Health (NIH) news release reported that a series of national epidemiological surveys on alcohol and related conditions found that DUD was more common among men, white and Native American individuals, and those who are single or no longer married. The surveys also reported that people with DUD were significantly more likely to have a broad range of psychiatric disorders, including mood, anxiety, PTSD, and personality disorders. Individuals with a DUD in the past year were 1.3 times as likely to experience clinical depression, 1.6 times as likely to have PTSD, and 1.8 times as likely to have borderline personality disorder than people without a DUD. Approximately 4% of Americans met the criteria for DUD in the previous year and about 10% have had DUD at some time in their lives (NIH, 2015).

Furthermore, according to the 2019 National Survey on Drug Use and Health (NSDUH), 14.5 million people ages 12 and older (5.3% of this age group) had AUD: 9.0 million men (6.8% of men in this age group) and 5.5 million women (3.9% of women in this age group). An estimated 95,000 people (approximately 68,000 men and 27,000 women) die from alcohol-related causes annually, making alcohol the third-leading preventable cause of death in the United States, after tobacco and poor diet/physical inactivity, respectively. Between 2011 and 2015, the leading causes of alcohol-attributable deaths due to chronic conditions in the United States were alcohol-associated liver disease, heart disease and stroke, unspecified liver cirrhosis, upper aerodigestive tract cancers, liver cancer, supraventricular cardiac dysrhythmia, breast cancer, and hypertension. In 2019, alcohol-impaired driving fatalities accounted for 10,142 deaths (28.0% of overall driving fatalities) (National Institutes of Alcohol Abuse and Alcoholism, 2021).

The DSM-5 eliminated the terms "abuse" and "dependence" that had been used in previous editions. Instead, it now uses a single disorder, which is rated by severity (mild, moderate, and severe; see Diagnostic Specifier below), depending on the number of symptoms met; individuals must meet at least two out of the listed symptoms within a 12-month period to be diagnosed with an SUD. Overall, the diagnosis of an SUD is based on a pathological pattern of behaviors, described below, which are related to use of the substance; each diagnosis, in turn, is associated with a substance class. There are ten classes of substances: (1) alcohol, (2) caffeine, (3) cannabis, (4) hallucinogens, (5) inhalants, (6) opioids, (7) sedatives, hypnotics, or anxiolytics, (8) stimulants, (9) tobacco, and (10) other (or unknown). In addition, the DSM-5 includes substance-induced disorders, such as intoxication and withdrawal. And other substance-/medication-induced mental disorders should always be considered in the evaluation of depression, anxiety, or psychosis, as underlying substance use is often present when psychiatric disorders do not respond to usual treatments (APA, 2013).

Overall, the diagnosis of an SUD is based on a pathological pattern of behaviors related to use of the substance. Table 2.19 presents the diagnostic criteria of SUD and the related pathological patterns of symptoms and behaviors under each criterion.

In addition to the diagnostic evaluation of substance-related disorders, there are many theories of the neurobiological basis of addiction resulting from the pathological hypersensitization of both drug-associated stimuli and drug-induced effects. Box 2.8 presents a summary of neurobiological theories of substance-related disorders, using alcohol as an example.

Table 2.19 Diagnostic Criteria of Pathological Pattern of Symptoms and Behaviors Related to Substance Use Disorder

Criteria	Criterion	Pathological Symptoms and Behaviors
1. Impaired control over substance use	1	Consumes the substance in a larger amount or over a longer period than originally intended
	2	Persistent desire to cut down or regulate substance use, and may report multiple unsuccessful efforts to decrease or discontinue it
	3	Spends a great deal of time obtaining the substance, using the substance, or recovering from its effects
	4	Cravings which manifest as an intense desire or urge for the substance and which may occur at any time but are more likely to occur when in an environment where the substance was previously obtained or used
2. Social impairment	5	Failure to fulfill major role obligations at work, school, or home
	6	Continued substance use despite having persistent or recurrent social or interpersonal problems
	7	Withdrawal from family activities and hobbies to use substance
3. Risky use of the substance	8	Recurrent substance use in situations in which it is physically hazardous
	9	Continued substance use despite knowledge of having a persistent or recurrent physical or psychological problem that is likely to have been caused or exacerbated by the substance
4. Pharmacological criteria	10	Tolerance signaled by requiring a markedly increased dose of the substance to achieve the desired effect or by a markedly reduced effect when the usual dose is consumed
	11	Withdrawal syndrome occurs when the concentrations of a substance decline in the body of an individual who had maintained prolonged heavy use of the substance; as a result, the individual is likely to consume the substance to relieve the symptoms

Source; Adapted from DSM-5, APA (2013).

Box 2.8 Neurobiological Bases of Substance-Related Disorders

Addiction is a psychiatric disorder. While there are many theories about the interactions between the neurobiological mechanisms of aberrant learning and memory behavior, it is strongly argued that addiction results from the pathological hypersensitization of both drug-associated stimuli and drug-induced effects. One pathway important to understanding the effects of drugs on the brain is called the reward pathway, which involves several parts of the brain: the ventral tegmental area (VTA), the nucleus accumbens (NA), and the prefrontal cortex.

For example, alcohol enhances dopamine release from the VTA to the NA and reduces glutamate excitotoxicity in the VTA. The positive reinforcing action of alcohol comes from the activation of the dopaminergic reward pathway in the limbic system:

1. When alcohol is consumed, dopamine is released in the VTA and projected to the NA, where it is acutely involved in motivation and reinforcement behaviors (alcohol craving).
2. Glutamate is the brain's major excitatory neurotransmitter system; alcohol reduces glutamate levels in the NA and suppresses glutamate-mediated signal transmission in the central nucleus of the amygdala.
3. Alcohol enhances dopamine release directly and indirectly through its interactions with GABAergic neurons and opioid receptors in the NAs.
4. GABA is the brain's major inhibitory neurotransmitter; alcohol enhances dopamine release from the VTA to the NA by disinhibiting GABA via endogenous opioids. The release of dopamine mediates alcohol's pleasurable and reinforcing actions.
5. Opioid systems involving endogenous opioids influence drinking behaviors via interaction with the mesolimbic system. Naltrexone is an opiate receptor antagonist that has been shown to limit cravings by reducing the positive reinforcement effect of alcohol consumption.
6. Psychologically, alcohol-seeking behavior is exacerbated by changes in the PFC, the region of the brain where decision-making and inhibitory control are governed.
7. Chronic exposure to alcohol progressively manipulates the PFC until decision-making and judging the consequences of one's actions become difficult.

Alcohol-Related Brain Involvement

The following key areas of the brain exhibit key neurofunctional abnormalities due to alcohol consumption:

1. Frontal lobes: Executive function, impaired judgment, impulsivity, blunted affect.
2. Hippocampus, thalamus/hypothalamus, and caudate callosum: Memory dysfunction.
3. Corpus callosum: Visuospatial abilities.
4. Corpus callosum and cerebellum: Upper and lower limb control.
5. Pons and cerebellum: Oculomotor control.

(Adapted from Stahl, 2013)

In this section, alcohol-related disorders are chosen as an example of how to conduct a mental status assessment and diagnostic evaluation, as they represent the classic condition in this group of disorders.

Diagnostic Criteria

DSM-5 Alcohol-Related Disorders Diagnostic Criteria Modified

The DSM-5 classifies alcohol-related disorders as (1) alcohol use disorder, (2) alcohol intoxication, (3) alcohol withdrawal, (4) other alcohol-induced disorder, and (5) unspecified alcohol-related disorder. Only alcohol use disorder, alcohol intoxication, and alcohol withdrawal are covered in this section, as other alcohol-induced disorder and unspecified alcohol-related disorder do not meet the full criteria for any specific alcohol-related disorder.

1. **Alcohol use disorder diagnostic criteria**

A. **Signs and Symptoms:** A pattern of alcohol use leading to clinically significant impairment or distress, as manifested by at least two of the following:

   1. Alcohol is often taken in larger amounts or over a longer period of time than intended.
   2. A persistent desire or unsuccessful efforts to cut down on or control alcohol use.
   3. A great deal of time is spent on activities necessary to obtain alcohol, use alcohol, or recover from its effects.
   4. Craving, or a strong desire or urge to use alcohol.
   5. Recurrent alcohol use that results in a failure to fulfill major role obligations at work, school, or home.
   6. Continued alcohol use despite having persistent or recurrent social or interpersonal problems caused or exacerbated by its effects.
   7. Important social, occupational, or recreational activities are given up or reduced because of alcohol use.
   8. Recurrent alcohol use in situations in which it is physically hazardous.
   9. Continued alcohol use despite knowledge of having a persistent or recurrent physical or psychological problem that is likely to have been caused or exacerbated by alcohol.
   10. Tolerance, as defined by either of the following:
       a. A need for markedly increased amounts of alcohol to achieve intoxication or the desired effect.
       b. A markedly diminished effect with continued use of the same amount of alcohol.
   11. Withdrawal, as manifested by either of the following:
       a. Characteristic withdrawal syndrome for alcohol (see the alcohol withdrawal diagnostic criteria listed below).
       b. Alcohol is taken to relieve or avoid withdrawal symptoms.

2. Alcohol intoxication diagnostic criteria

A. Recent ingestion of alcohol.

B. Clinically significant problematic behavioral or psychological changes (e.g., inappropriate sexual or aggressive behavior, mood lability, impaired judgment, impaired social or occupational functioning) that develop during, or shortly after, ingestion of alcohol.

C. **Signs and Symptoms:** One or more of the following signs or symptoms developing during or shortly after alcohol ingestion:

1. Slurred speech.
2. Incoordination.
3. Unsteady gait.
4. Nystagmus.
5. Impairment in attention or memory.
6. Stupor or coma.

D. The signs or symptoms are not attributable to another medical condition (e.g., diabetic ketoacidosis) and are not better explained by another mental disorder (e.g., delirium), including intoxication with another substance (e.g., benzodiazepines).

E. **Associated Features Supporting Alcohol Intoxication Diagnosis:** Alcohol intoxication is sometimes associated with amnesia of the events that occurred during the course of the intoxication ("blackouts").

F. **Coding Note:** Coding for alcohol intoxication depends on whether there is a comorbid alcohol use disorder. If alcohol use disorder is comorbid, severity specifiers (mild, moderate, or severe) are required.

3. Alcohol withdrawal diagnostic criteria

A. Cessation of (or reduction) in alcohol use that has been heavy and prolonged.

B. **Signs and Symptoms:** Two (or more) of the following symptoms developing within several hours to a few days after cessation of (or reduction in) alcohol use:

1. Autonomic hyperactivity (e.g., sweating or pulse rate greater than 100 bpm).
2. Increased hand tremor.
3. Insomnia.
4. Nausea or vomiting.
5. Transient visual, tactile, or auditory hallucinations or illusions.
6. Psychomotor agitation.
7. Anxiety.
8. Generalized tonic-clonic seizures.

C.   The signs or symptoms in Criterion B lead to clinically significant distress or impairment in social, occupational, or other important areas of functioning.

D.   The signs or symptoms are not attributable to another medical condition and are not better explained by another mental disorder, including intoxication or withdrawal from another substance.

E.   **Diagnostic Specifier:**
     With perceptual disturbances: This specifier applies when hallucinations (usually visual or tactile) occur with intact reality testing, or when auditory, visual, or tactile illusions occur in the absence of delirium.
     Current severity:

     Mild: Presence of two or three symptoms.
     Moderate: Presence of four or five symptoms.
     Severe: Presence of six or more symptoms.

F.   **Associated Features Supporting Diagnosis:** Alcohol withdrawal delirium tremens with symptoms of altered consciousness, confusion, agitation, cognitive impairment, and visual, tactile, and, rarely, auditory hallucinations.

G.   **Coding Note:** Alcohol withdrawal can only occur in the presence of a moderate or severe alcohol use disorder. Therefore, it is not permissible to code a comorbid mild alcohol use disorder with alcohol withdrawal.

Interviewing Techniques in Assessment of Alcohol Use Disorder

The following samples of diagnostic interview questions are provided as guidelines to help the APMHN to elicit the symptoms of alcohol use disorder and alcohol intoxication during the initial client psychiatric evaluation. Each question is outlined based on the diagnostic criteria following the client's clinical presentation, information obtained from others, and the clinician's observations (adopted from NIH–NIAAA, December, 2020).

1. Alcohol Use Disorder Diagnostic Criteria

A. Signs and Symptoms: A problematic pattern of alcohol use leading to clinically significant impairment or distress, as manifested by at least two of the following:

1.   Alcohol is often taken in larger amounts or over a longer period than was intended.
     Question: *In the past year, have you had times when you ended up drinking more, or longer, than you intended?*
2.   There is a persistent desire or unsuccessful effort to cut down on or control alcohol use.
     Question: *In the past year, have you more than once wanted to cut down on or to stop drinking, or tried to do so but couldn't?*

3. A great deal of time is spent on activities necessary to obtain alcohol, use alcohol, or recover from its effects.

   Question: *In the past year, have you spent a lot of time drinking? Or being sick or getting over the aftereffects of drinking?*

4. Craving, or a strong desire or urge to use alcohol.

   Question: *In the past year, have you wanted a drink so badly you couldn't think of anything else?*

5. Recurrent alcohol use that results in failure to fulfill major role obligations at work, school, or home.

   Question: *In the past year, have you found that drinking—or being sick from drinking—often interfered with taking care of your home or family? Or caused job troubles? Or school problems?*

6. Continued alcohol use despite having persistent or recurrent social or inter-personal problems caused or exacerbated by the effects of alcohol.

   Question: *In the past year, have you continued to drink even though it was causing trouble with your family or friends?*

7. Important social, occupational, or recreational activities are given up or reduced because of alcohol use.

   Question: *In the past year, have you given up or cut back on activities that were important or interesting to you, or that gave you pleasure, in order to drink?*

8. Recurrent alcohol use in situations in which it is physically hazardous.

   Question: *In the past year, have you more than once gotten into situations while or after drinking that increased your chances of getting hurt (such as driving, swimming, using machinery, walking in a dangerous area, or having unprotected sex)?*

9. Alcohol use is continued despite knowledge of having a persistent or recur-rent physical or psychological problem that is likely to have been caused or exacerbated by alcohol.

   Question: *In the past year, have you continued to drink even though it was making you feel depressed or anxious or adding to another health problem? Or after having had a memory blackout?*

10. Tolerance, as defined by either of the following:

    a. A need for markedly increased amounts of alcohol to achieve intoxica-tion or the desired effect.

    b. A markedly diminished effect with continued use of the same amount of alcohol.

       Question: *In the past year, have you had to drink more than you once did to get the effect you want? Or have you found that your usual number of drinks had much less of an effect than before?*

11. Withdrawal, as manifested by either of the following:

    a. The characteristic withdrawal syndrome for alcohol (see alcohol with-drawal diagnostic criteria).

    b. Alcohol is taken to relieve or avoid withdrawal symptoms.

Question: *In the past year, have you found that when the effects of alcohol were wearing off, you had withdrawal symptoms, such as trouble sleeping, shakiness, restlessness, nausea, sweating, a racing heart, or a seizure? Or sensed things that were not there?*

2. Alcohol Intoxication Diagnostic Criteria

1. **Recent ingestion of alcohol:**
   Question: *When was the last time you had a drink and how much was it?*
2. **Clinically significant problematic behavioral or psychological changes:**
   Information obtained from others: *The husband reported the client's inability to care for herself and children, marital problems, anxiety disorder.*

A. **Signs and Symptoms:** One or more of the following signs or symptoms developing during or shortly after alcohol use:

   1. Slurred speech.
   2. Incoordination.
   3. Unsteady gait.
   4. Nystagmus.
   5. Impairment in attention or memory.
   6. Stupor or coma.

The following presents a case exemplar of the initial psychiatric evaluation, including how the diagnosis of alcohol intoxication with comorbid alcohol use disorder is determined, along with rationales.

Case Exemplar

A. *Identification, Chief Complaint, and Reason for Referral*

The client is a 57-year-old white, married female brought to the ER by the emergency medical services (EMS). She was accompanied by her husband, who found her face down on the front deck of the house when he came home from work. Upon arrival at the hospital, she appeared to be lethargic, disoriented, and to have slurred speech, but responded when her name was called. When she was asked what brought her to the hospital, she said, "I have been drinking."

B. *History of Present Illness*

The client reported that for the last several months, she has been suffering from insomnia, awakening frequently during the night, and has had a poor appetite, resulting in a 35 lb weight loss in 3 months. She was vague about her drinking patterns prior to experiencing these symptoms, but claimed that over the past 2 weeks, her drinking has increased rapidly from a bottle of wine at night to help her sleep to two bottles of wine and a quarter of a 750-mL bottle of vodka throughout the day. She was unable to get up most mornings on time to get herself ready to go to work, resulting in frequent lateness to or absence from work.

This morning, prior to arrival to the ER, she had three drinks of vodka instead of breakfast before passing out. She was not sure of the exact time of her last drink. During the interview, the client was anxious, irritable, had difficulty sitting still, and both hands were tremulous, indicating that she is transitioning from alcohol intoxication to withdrawal. The APMHN decided to admit the client to the intensive care unit (ICU) for observation of potentially serious alcohol withdrawal and to begin an alcohol detoxification regimen intervention. Additional pertinent information was obtained from the client's husband, and the client will be followed up the next day for additional information while in the hospital.

C. *Past Psychiatric History*

According to the client's husband, the client has a history of depression, anxiety, and alcohol use disorder, dating back 30 years. For 2 years, she was treated effectively with sedatives, antidepressants, and biweekly psychotherapy, but she stopped both the medications and therapy 2 years ago. Since then, she has had a long period of social drinking. Over the last year, her drinking has increased from an average of eight or nine drinks per week to one or two bottles of wine and at least four drinks of vodka a day. Three months ago, she was admitted to the hospital ICU for 3 days due to a fainting episode following heavy drinking, and against medical advice she discharged herself. Since then, she has resumed drinking and has refused to get any help, claiming that she could control her drinking by cutting down. The client has no history of alcohol-related delirium, seizures, or hallucinations, but has had several "blackout" episodes. She has no history of psychiatric hospitalization, and no past history of suicidal gestures or attempts.

The following information is obtained from the second interview, which was conducted the next day in the ICU.

D. *Substance Use History*

The client reported:
1. A history of using marijuana on a weekly basis for about 5 years in her early 20s.
2. Using cocaine once when she was in high school.
3. Smoking half a pack of cigarettes a day for the last 30 years.
4. Beginning to drink alcohol socially at the age of 17, when she went out with friends, and her drinking increased in her 20s. She has had significant alcohol intake in the past year and required a brief admission to the ICU for stabilization. She has had a persistent desire to cut down but has been unsuccessful, as her cravings for alcohol are so powerful that each time she tried to stop she always gave in. She denies other substance use.

E. *Psychosocial and Developmental History*

1. *Education*: The client has an associate's degree in liberal science.
2. *Family Relationships, Social Network, and Abuse History*: The client is an only child. Both parents are alive, but she is estranged from them due

to her drinking issues. She is married with no children. Marital conflict due to her drinking has progressively worsened; for the last month, she and her husband have been sleeping in separate rooms. She stated that her husband has been very supportive and patient with her until now and told her that he did not want to be with her unless she got help. She has lost most of her close friends, including her drinking partners, since her drinking got out of control. No abuse or maltreatment history reported.

3. *Employment Record*: The client works as a teacher's aide at an elementary school. As of now, her work is in jeopardy due to her frequent lateness and absences.
4. *Legal Record*: No legal issues reported. She claimed that she never got a DWI (driving while intoxicated).
5. *Religious Background*: The client reported that she is not religious, but was raised Catholic.

F. *Family Mental Health History*

Father has a history of substance use, mostly alcohol, but stopped drinking 10 years ago when he was threatened by her mother, who filed for divorce. No known psychiatric illness and treatment reported.

G. *Review of Systems*

See the medical record, as the client has been undergoing a full medical workup, including laboratory tests. She has started a detoxification regimen with librium and additional supplements: folic acid 1 mg po daily and thiamine 100 mg po daily. During the interview, she exhibited no visual signs of distress, including no symptoms of alcohol withdrawal, and appeared to be responding well to the detoxification regimen.

H. *Mental Status Examination*

1. *Appearance and Behavior*: The client appeared to be the stated age, wearing a hospital gown. She was cooperative with the interview, making good eye contact, occasionally became tearful while talking about her past histories.
2. *Mood*: Sad and depressed.
3. *Affect*: Guarded, tearful, and constricted.
4. *Thought Content and Process*: Speech: Soft tone of voice, rate and volume within normal limits, and goal directed. Thought process: Rational and logical; no looseness of associations, tangential thoughts, or thought blocking. No evidence of delusional thoughts.
5. *Perceptual Disturbances*: She denies auditory/visual/tactile hallucinations, or illusions.
6. *Sensorium, Cognitive, and Intellectual Functioning*: Alert and oriented × 3. She is fully aware of her drinking problem and its impact on her life, and is seriously considering getting help after discharge from the hospital.

I. *Diagnosis and Treatment Plan*

1. **DSM-5 Diagnosis:** Alcohol intoxication, alcohol use disorder.

2. ***Rationale for Diagnostic Impression***: According to the DSM-5 (APA, 2013), the following criteria must be present to diagnose alcohol intoxication. The client meets those criteria, as indicated by the bold symptom categories and the client's clinical presentations:

A. ***Recent ingestion of alcohol.*** The client drank "three drinks of vodka" instead of having breakfast this morning, and then passed out.

B. Clinically significant ***problematic behavioral or psychological changes.*** As a result of her drinking, she has suffered with depression and anxiety, and her marriage and job are in serious trouble.

C. **Signs and Symptoms:** One or more of the following signs or symptoms developing during or shortly after alcohol use:

   1. Slurred speech.
   2. Incoordination.
   3. Unsteady gait.
   4. Nystagmus.
   5. Impairment in attention or memory.
   6. Stupor or coma.

   Prior to visiting the hospital ER, the client was found unconscious by her husband. At the time of the first interview, the client presented with symptoms of lethargy, unsteady gait, disorientation, and slurred speech (Criteria C1, 2, 5, and 6).

D. The signs or symptoms are ***not attributable to another medical condition*** and are not better explained by another mental disorder, including intoxication with another substance. The client and the husband denied that the client had been diagnosed with any medical or psychiatric conditions, and also denied that she was abusing any other substances.

E. **Associated Features Supporting Alcohol Intoxication Diagnosis:** Alcohol intoxication is sometimes associated with amnesia of the events that occurred during the course of the intoxication ("blackouts"). The client admitted experiencing blackouts.

F. **Coding Note:** Coding for alcohol intoxication depends on whether there is a comorbid alcohol use disorder. If there is, severity specifiers (mild, moderate, or severe) are required.

In addition to alcohol intoxication, the client also meets the diagnostic criteria of alcohol use disorder, as indicated below by the bold symptom categories and the associated client's clinical presentations.

A. **Signs and Symptoms:** A problematic pattern of alcohol use leading to clinically significant impairment or distress, as manifested by at least two of the following:

   1. Alcohol is often taken in larger amounts or over a longer period than was intended.
      The client's social drinking of alcohol started at the age of 17, when she went out with friends, and increased in her 20s. She has had

significant alcohol intake in the past year and required a brief admission to the ICU for stabilization.

2. There is a persistent desire or unsuccessful efforts to cut down on or control alcohol use.

    The client has had the persistent desire to cut down on her drinking but has been unsuccessful.

3. A great deal of time is spent on activities necessary to obtain alcohol, use alcohol, or recover from its effects.

4. Craving, or a strong desire or urge to use alcohol.

    The client's cravings for alcohol are so powerful that each time she tried to stop she always gave in.

5. Recurrent alcohol use, resulting in a failure to fulfill major role obligations at work, school, or home.

    The client's job is in jeopardy due to her frequent lateness and absences as a result of her drinking.

6. Continued alcohol use despite persistent or recurrent social or interpersonal problems caused or exacerbated by the effects of alcohol.

    The client's marriage has been in jeopardy, as her husband gave her an ultimatum whether to get help or to separate. She has lost all of her friends and is estranged from her parents due to her drinking issues.

7. Important social, occupational, or recreational activities are given up or reduced because of alcohol use.

8. Recurrent alcohol use in situations in which it is physically hazardous.

    The client minimizes the impact of her alcohol intake on her physical health. Laboratory findings and test results are still pending. The client admitted several episodes of "blackouts."

9. Alcohol use is continued despite knowledge of having a persistent or recurrent physical or psychological problem that is likely to have been caused or exacerbated by alcohol.

    During the second interview, the client showed significant mood disturbances of sadness, anxiety, and depressed mood, suggesting that her drinking exacerbated these symptoms.

10. Tolerance, as defined by either of the following:

    a. A need for markedly increased amounts of alcohol to achieve intoxication or desired effect.

    The client admitted that her drinking has increased during the last year, from an average of eight or nine drinks per week to one or two bottles of wine and at least four drinks of vodka a day.

    b. A markedly diminished effect with continued use of the same amount of alcohol.

11. Withdrawal, as manifested by either of the following:

    a. The characteristic withdrawal syndrome for alcohol (see the alcohol withdrawal diagnostic criteria).

    b. Alcohol is taken to relieve or avoid withdrawal symptoms.

B. **Duration:** A problematic pattern of alcohol use leading to clinically significant impairment or distress occurring within a 12-month period.

The client's drinking increased in her 20s. She has also had a significant increase in alcohol intake in the past year and required a brief admission to the ICU for stabilization.

C. **Current Severity Specifiers:**

Mild: Presence of two or three symptoms.

Moderate: Presence of four or five symptoms.

Severe: Presence of six or more symptoms.

The client met a total of 8 out of 11 symptom criteria, which indicates the severity specifier of "severe."

Final diagnosis is confirmed as alcohol intoxication with comorbid alcohol use disorder—severe.

3. *Treatment Plan and Summary*:

Treatment Plan:

- Stabilize the client medically while in ICU.
- Upon discharge from ICU, recommend that the client continues alcohol rehabilitation at a designated facility.
- Since the client has a history of anxiety and depression in addition to alcohol use disorder, further evaluation is recommended for comorbid psychiatric disorders (e.g., anxiety disorder and depressive disorder) vs. alcohol-induced psychiatric disorders.

Summary: The client is a 57-year-old white, married female brought to the ER by EMS, accompanied by her husband, who found her unconscious and called 911. Upon arrival at the hospital, the client appeared to be lethargic, disoriented, with slurred speech, but responded when her name was called. The client had a strong alcohol breath and the APMHN suspected that she was intoxicated with alcohol. As the interview progressed, the APMHN found her to be more alert and able to respond to questions, but the client also became anxious and irritable, with bilateral hand tremors. The APMHN determined that the client was transitioning from alcohol intoxication to alcohol withdrawal, as her last drink was approximately 8 hours ago, and decided to admit the client to the intensive care unit for medical evaluation and alcohol detoxification treatment. The next day, the APMHN followed up with the client in the ICU to complete the initial psychiatric evaluation and determined a diagnosis of alcohol intoxication with comorbid alcohol use disorder—severe.

As noted earlier, alcohol-related medical complications are the leading causes of alcohol-attributable deaths—for example, alcohol-associated liver disease, heart disease and stroke, unspecified liver cirrhosis, upper aerodigestive tract cancers, liver cancer, supraventricular cardiac dysrhythmia, and hypertension. Table 2.20 presents the list of laboratory tests for the APMHN to order to rule out each related disease.

Table 2.20 Alcohol and Its Medical Complications

Medical Complication	Abnormal Lab Findings of ETOH Use Disorder

• Gastritis or gastric ulcers
• Pancreatitis
• Esophagitis
• Hypertension
• Cardiomyopathy arrhythmias
• Alcoholic hepatitis
• Liver cirrhosis
• High risk of cancer in all affected areas
	• Blood alcohol level (>100 mg/dL)
	• Elevated
	  • Mean corpuscular volume (MCV)
	  • Gamma-glutamyl transferase (GGT)
	  • Aspartate aminotransferase (AST)
	  • Alanine aminotransferase (ALT)
	• Elevated amylase
	• Low Na (sodium) and K (potassium)
	• Elevated serum lipids
	• Elevated uric acid and triglycerides
	• Decreased WBC, granulocyte, and thrombocytopenia

Section 9: Neurocognitive Disorders

Neurocognitive disorders (NCDs) are unique among DSM-5 categories in that there are NCD syndromes (e.g., major, mild), as well as NCDs due to underlying disease entities (e.g., NCD due to Alzheimer's disease [AD]) (APA, 2013). Sadock et al. (2019) classify major NCDs into one of three conditions: (1) delirium, (2) dementia, and (3) other cognitive disorders. However, the DSM-5 no longer uses the term "dementia" as a diagnosis, but instead uses NCD with etiological subtypes (e.g., AD, frontotemporal lobar degeneration, Lewy body disease, and vascular disease). All criteria for NCDs are based upon defined cognitive domains.

Delirium develops over a short period of time (usually hours to a few days) with acute onset of fluctuating cognitive impairment, and a disturbance of consciousness. Delirium is a syndrome, not a disease. It is a common disorder among the elderly (13% in the general population age 85 years and older). The highest rate of hospital-based delirium is found in post-cardiotomy patients (more than 90% in some studies); in addition, approximately 30% of open-heart surgery patients, 20% of severe burn patients, and 30–40% of hospitalized patients with acquired immune deficiency syndrome were reported to have delirium (Sadock et al., 2019).

The prevalence of moderate to severe NCD with etiological subtypes is approximately 5% in the general population older than 65 years of age, and 20–40% in the general population older than 85 years of age. NCD due to AD is the most common, accounting for 50–60% of NCDs. It affects as many as 5% of persons over age 65, and 15–20% of persons age 85 or older. Risk factors include being female and having a first-degree relative with the disorder. There are two types of NCD due to AD: early onset (onset before or at age 65) and late onset (onset after age 65). Onset is usually initially insidious, and slowly becomes progressive. After several years, aphasia, apraxia, and agnosia often became apparent, and in later stages motor and gait disturbances may develop to the point where the person is bedridden. Mean survival is 8 years, with a range from 1 to 20 years; the earlier the onset, the longer the mean survival rate. Another common subtype of NCD is vascular dementia, which is commonly caused by cerebrovascular diseases and ranges from 0.2% in the 65–70 years age group to 16% in individuals 80 years and older (Sadock et al., 2019; APA, 2013).

NCD with etiological subtypes and delirium have some common features, and differentiating between the two diagnoses requires knowing the characteristic features of each, as well as establishing the client's premorbid cognitive status by obtaining a client history and conducting cognitive and delirium screens (see Table 2.21).

The core feature of NCDs is acquired cognitive decline in one or more cognitive domains (see Table 2.22) based on (1) a concern about cognition on the part of the individual, a knowledgeable informant, or the clinician; and (2) performance on an objective assessment that falls below the expected level or that has been observed to decline over time. Table 2.22 provides a brief summary of cognitive domains and the required symptoms in one (or more) of them to diagnose major and mild NCDs (see the DSM-5, pp. 593–595, for more detailed information).

These cognitive impairments are frequently complicated by behavioral symptoms of disorientation, poor judgment, inability to form an interpersonal relationship, and lack of problem-solving abilities.

Table 2.23 shows the etiological subtype specifier differentiating between degenerative and nondegenerative types of NCDs.

Table 2.21 Differential Diagnostic Features between NCD with Etiological Subtypes and Delirium

Feature	NCD with Etiological Subtypes (commonly known as dementia)	Delirium
Onset	Slow and insidious onset	Sudden onset; over hours or days
Duration	Months to years	Hours or weeks, but can be longer
Course	Symptoms are progressive over a long period of time; not reversible	Short and fluctuating; often worse at night and on waking; usually reversible with treatment of the underlying condition
Alertness	Generally normal	Can fluctuate from hypervigilant to very lethargic
Attention	Preserved and generally normal	Impaired or fluctuates, difficulty following conversation
Memory	Impaired remote memory	Impaired recent and immediate memory
Speech	Difficulty with word finding	Incoherent (slow or rapid)
Thoughts	Difficulty with word finding	Disorganized, distorted, fragmented
Psychomotor activity	• Wandering/exit seeking • Agitated or withdrawn	• Hyperactive delirium: Agitation, restlessness, hallucinations • Hypoactive delirium: Sleepy, slow moving • Mixed: Alternating features of above
Perception	Usually absent except NCD due to Lewy body	Distorted: Illusions, hallucinations, delusions; difficulty distinguishing between reality and misperceptions

Source: Adapted from Victoria Department of Hospital & Health Services (2021).

Table 2.22 Neurocognitive Domain and Symptom Examples

Cognitive Domain	Symptom Examples
1. Complex attention (sustained attention, divided attention, selective attention, processing speed)	*Major:* Difficulty in environments with multiple stimuli, holding new information, unable to perform mental calculation, all thinking takes longer than usual *Minor:* Normal tasks take longer than previously, finding errors in routine tasks, needs more double-checking, thinking is easier when not with multiple stimuli
2. Executive function (planning, decision-making, working memory, responding to feedback/error correction, overriding habits/inhibition, mental flexibility)	*Major:* Needs to focus on one task at a time, needs to rely on others to plan instrumental activities of daily living or make decisions *Minor:* Requires extra effort to complete multistage projects, organize/plan/make decisions, and follow shifting conversation in social setting; difficulty resuming a task once interrupted
3. Learning/memory (immediate memory, recent memory [including recall, cued recall, and recognition memory], very-long term memory [sematic; autobiographical], implicit learning)	*Major:* Repeats self within the same conversation, unable to keep track of short list of items when shopping or of plans for the day, needs a frequent reminder to orient to task at hand *Minor:* Difficulty recalling recent events, relies on list making or calendar, re-reading to keep track of characters in a movie or novel, repeats self over a few weeks to the same person, loses track of whether or not bills have already been paid
4. Language (expressive language [including naming, word finding, fluency, and grammar and syntax] and receptive language)	*Major:* Significant difficulties with expressive or receptive language, uses general-use phrases such as "that thing" and "you know what I mean," with severe impairment may not recall names of close friends and family; echolalia and automatic speech typically precede mutism *Minor:* Noticeable word-finding difficulty; may substitute general for specific terms, avoid use of specific names of acquaintances, grammatical errors involving subtle omission or incorrect use of articles, prepositions, auxiliary verbs, etc.
5. Perceptual-motor (includes abilities subsumed under the terms: *visual perception, visuo-constructional perceptual-motor, praxis, and gnosis*)	*Major:* Significant difficulties with previously familiar activities, navigating in familiar environments, often more confused at dusk *Minor:* Needs to rely more on maps or others for directions, uses notes and follows others to get to a new place, finds self lost or turned around when not concentrating on task, less precise in parking, needs to expend greater effort for spatial tasks, such as carpentry, assembly, sewing, or knitting
6. Social cognition (recognition of emotions, theory of mind)	*Major:* Behavior clearly out of acceptable social range, focuses excessively on a topic despite groups' disinterest or direct feedback, makes decisions without regard to safety, typically has little insight into own behaviors *Minor:* Subtle changes in behavior or attitude, often described as a change in personality, less ability to recognize social cues or read facial expressions, decreased empathy, increased extraversion or introversion, decreased inhibition, or subtle or episodic apathy or restlessness

Table 2.23 Etiological Subtype Specifier: Degenerative vs. Nondegenerative Types

Degenerative NCDs	*Nondegenerative NCDs*
Alzheimer's disease	Vascular disease
Frontotemporal lobar degermation	Traumatic brain injury
Lewy body disease	Substance/medication induced
Parkinson's disease	HIV infection
Huntington's disease	

Source: Adapted from Sadock et al. (2019).

In addition to etiological subtype specifiers, behavioral disturbance is another important specifier for a final NCD diagnosis—that is, either with or without behavioral disturbance. Specifier: (1) *without behavioral disturbance* if the cognitive disturbance is not accompanied by any clinically significant behavioral disturbance, such as psychotic symptoms, mood disturbance, agitation, apathy, or other behavioral symptoms; (2) *with behavioral disturbance* if the cognitive disturbance is accompanied by a clinically significant behavioral disturbance (APA, 2013).

NCDs differ from age-associated memory impairment (normal aging), which presents as a decreased ability to learn new material, a slowing of thought processes, and benign senescent forgetfulness. In addition, memory impairment due to normal aging does not show a progressive deteriorating course, as seen in NCDs. Similarly, another common psychiatric illness—depression in the elderly—may also present as cognitive impairment or as a comorbid illness with NCD. It is therefore critically important to conduct a careful assessment with cognitive screening to rule out possible treatable causes, as well as to provide a baseline to differentiate whether the decline in cognition is due to depression, for example, or to NCD. The most commonly used cognitive assessment tools are the Standardized Mini-Mental State Examination (SMMSE), the Abbreviated Mental Test Score (AMTS), and the Clock Drawing Test (CDT) (Victoria Department of Hospital & Health Services, 2021).

Diagnostic Criteria

In this section, neurocognitive disorder due to AD is chosen as an example to address the diagnostic evaluations of NCDs, as it is the most common cause of NCDs and represents the classic condition in this group of disorders.

DSM-5 Criteria for Major or Mild Neurocognitive Disorder due to AD Modified

A. The criteria are met for major or mild neurocognitive disorder (see Table 2.24).
B. There is insidious onset and gradual progression of impairment in one or more cognitive domains (see Table 2.22; for major neurocognitive disorder, at least two domains must be impaired).
C. Criteria are met for either probable or possible AD as shown in Table 2.25.

Table 2.24 DSM-5 Modified Diagnostic Criteria for Major and Mild Neurocognitive Disorders

Major Neurocognitive Disorder	Mild Neurocognitive Disorder
A. Evidence of significant cognitive decline from a previous level of performance in one or more cognitive domains (see Table 2.22) based on A1 and A2:	
A1. Concern of the individual, a knowledgeable informant, or the clinician that there has been a significant decline in cognitive function; and	Concern of the individual, a knowledgeable informant, or the clinician that there has been a mild decline in cognitive function; and
A2. A substantial impairment in cognitive performance, preferably documented by standardized neuropsychological testing or, in its absence, another quantified clinical assessment.	A modest impairment in cognitive performance, preferably documented by standardized neuropsychological testing or, in its absence, another quantified clinical assessment.
B. The cognitive deficits interfere with independence in everyday activities (i.e., at a minimum, requiring assistance with complex instrumental activities of daily living, such as paying bills or managing medications).	The cognitive deficits do not interfere with capacity for independence in everyday activities (i.e., complex instrumental activities of daily living, such as paying bills or managing medications are preserved, but greater effort, compensatory strategies, or accommodations may be required).
C. The cognitive deficits do not occur exclusively in the context of a delirium.	
D. The cognitive deficits are not better explained by a mental disorder (e.g., major depressive disorder, schizophrenia).	

Source: Adapted from DSM-5, APA (2013).

D. The disturbance is not better explained by cerebrovascular disease, another neurodegenerative disease, the effects of a substance or of another mental, neurological, or systemic disorder.

Diagnostic note example: "Probable (possible) major (minor) neurocognitive disorder due to AD with (without) behavioral disturbance."

For early-onset cases with autosomal dominant inheritance, a mutation in one of the known causative AD genes—amyloid precursor protein (APP), presenilin 1 (PSEN1), or presenilin 2 (PSEN2)—may be involved, and genetic testing for such mutations is commercially available for PSEN1. At present, various biomarkers related to AD are identified, but not fully validated, and many are available only in tertiary care settings (Sadock et al., 2019).

Diagnostic markers for AD are based on the hallmarks of the following pathological findings and may have diagnostic value:

1. Diffuse cortical atrophy and enlarged ventricle detected on CT or MRI, and decreased brain acetylcholine metabolism.
2. Amyloid-based diagnostic test, such as amyloid imaging or brain positron emission tomography scan.

Table 2.25 Differentiation between Major and Minor Neurocognitive Disorder due to Alzheimer's disease (AD)

Major Neurocognitive Disorder due to AD	*Minor Neurocognitive Disorder due to AD*

Probable AD is diagnosed if either of the following is present; otherwise, possible AD should be diagnosed:
 	
1. Evidence of a causative AD genetic mutation from family history or genetic testing; or
2. All three of the following are present:
  a. Clear evidence of decline in memory and learning, and at least one other cognitive domain (based on detailed history or serial neuropsychological testing).
  b. Steadily progressive, gradual decline in cognition, without extended plateaus.
  c. No evidence of mixed etiology (i.e., absence of another neurogenerative or cerebrovascular disease, or another neurological, mental, or systematic disease or condition that is likely contributing to cognitive decline).
	Possible AD is diagnosed if all three of the following are present:
	Clear evidence of decline in memory and learning.
	Steadily progressive, gradual decline in cognition, without extended plateaus.
	No evidence of mixed etiology (i.e., absence of another neurogenerative or cerebrovascular disease, or another neurological or systematic disease or condition that may contribute to cognitive decline).

3. Reduced levels of amyloid beta-42 in the cerebrospinal fluid (CSF) (Table 2.26).

Table 2.26 Pathological and Clinical Features of Degenerative Neurocognitive Disorders

Disorder	*Pathology*	*Clinical Features*
Alzheimer's disease	Amyloid/tau pathology	Memory deficit Aphasia Apraxia Agnosia
NCD with Lewy bodies	Alpha-synuclein pathology	Memory deficit Fluctuating attention Extrapyramidal signs Psychosis (well-formed and detailed visual hallucinations)
Frontotemporal NCD	Tau pathology	Memory deficit Speech/language disorders Behavioral disinhibition Hyperorality Aphasia or inertia
Huntington's disease	Trinucleotide repeat	Memory deficit Executive dysfunction Chorea

(Continued)

Table 2.26 Continued

Disorder	Pathology	Clinical Features
Prion disease	Abnormal isoform of a cellular glycoprotein (Prion protein)	Memory deficit Ataxia Myoclonus Language disturbance
Parkinson's disease	Alpha-synuclein pathology	Cognitive decline Apathy Depressed and anxious mood Hallucinations/delusions Personality changes Rapid eye movement sleep behavior Excessive daytime sleep

Source: Adapted from Stahl (2013).

Interviewing Techniques in Assessment of Neurocognitive Disorder due to AD

Six components of a diagnostic evaluation enable the APMHN to obtain the information necessary to assess a client with potential NCD due to AD: (1) interviewing the client to take a history, (2) interviewing a caregiver or family member, (3) physical examination, (4) brief cognitive tests, (5) laboratory tests, and (6) structural imaging tests, if indicated.

The interview process with an individual with NCD due to AD can be challenging because one of its hallmark symptoms, along with memory loss, is difficulty expressing thoughts (such as in word-finding problems) or in understanding them (often called receptive communication). Basic effective communication strategies when assessing a client with NCD due to AD for diagnostic evaluation would be helpful not only for the clinician but also for the caregiver(s) of the person.

Engaging in therapeutic communication with respect and genuine warmth is a basic rule to increase the odds of successfully engaging in a diagnostic assessment interview, whether or not the client has an NCD; however, it is even more important for a person with NCD due to AD. Heerema (2019) highlighted nine tips when talking with a client who may have NCD due to AD:

1. *Don't Infantilize the Person*: Don't talk down to the person or treat them like an infant. Regardless of how much the person with NCD due to AD can or cannot understand, treat the person with honor and use a respectful tone of voice.
2. *Use Their Names and Preferred Titles*: Learn what the person's preferred name is and use it. Avoid using "honey," "sweetheart," or similar terms. You may mean it genuinely in affection, but it can also come across as demeaning or patronizing.
3. *Use Gentle Touch*: Knowing how someone responds to physical touch is important. While some people might get defensive if their personal space is invaded, many appreciate a gentle touch, such as giving a little pat on the shoulder or holding their hand while talking with them. Personal touch is important and can be an effective way to communicate that you care.

4. *Don't Just Talk Loudly*: Not every person with NCD due to AD has a hearing impairment and using a loud tone can make the individual feel like you are yelling at them. Use a clear, normal tone of voice to start a conversation unless the person has a hearing problem. Then adjust the volume as needed.

5. *Don't Use Slang or Figures of Speech*: As NCD due to AD progresses, it can become harder for the person to understand what is said to them. For example, telling the person with NCD due to AD that it's "no use crying over spilled milk" might result in them looking to see where the milk has spilled, rather than understanding the meaning of the proverb. In fact, the proverb interpretation test, which asks the test taker to interpret abstract ideas, such as the spilled milk reference above, is one way to screen for symptoms of NCD due to AD.

6. *Don't Ignore the Person*: When asking a question to the client with NCD due to AD, first give them a chance to respond before turning to the family member or caregiver for an answer. Also, don't talk about the person as if they're not there. They might understand more than the interviewer gives them credit for, so convey the respect by addressing them directly.

7. *Position Yourself at Their Level*: Rather than standing up straight and looking down at someone who may be seated, bend down to be at their level. This might make the interviewer less comfortable physically, but it will facilitate a more comfortable and respectful conversation.

8. *Avoid Interrogating*: Limit the questions to a small number, as the interviewer's goal is to provide encouragement during the visit, not to fire endless questions at the client that may be difficult to answer and that may potentially overwhelm the client.

9. *Smile and Make Eye Contact*: A genuine smile can reduce the chance of challenging behaviors since the client may feel reassured by the interviewer's nonverbal communication. A warm smile and eye contact convey that the interviewer is glad to be with the client and are highly important factors in therapeutic communications.

The following is a sample case exemplar of the initial psychiatric evaluation of a person with NCD, including how the diagnosis of NCD due to AD is determined, with the rationales and treatment plan.

Case Exemplar

The client's initials are KK.

A. *Identification, Chief Complaint, and Reason for Referral*

KK is a 76-year-old married, Caribbean-American male, referred by his primary care provider for a full psychiatric evaluation for potential NCD (dementia). KK was brought to the clinic by his wife with the chief complaint of, "I get confused a lot and I don't remember where I am at times, and I find it difficult to remember if I have paid my bills." He is alert and oriented to person and place, but unable to identify the current date. KK presents with a flat affect, but is cooperative with the assessment. Most of the information was received from his wife, who is his primary caregiver, due to the client's inability to answer most of the questions. A Mini-Mental Status Examination (MMSE) was conducted and KK scored 10 out of 30, indicating moderate cognitive impairment.

B. *History of Present Illness*

KK's wife reported that KK has had a long period of forgetfulness starting about a year ago, when he would forget where he placed the keys and at times would forget driving directions to the house where they have lived for over 30 years. KK periodically asks his wife if they have children and grandchildren. He often does not remember the current date and often asks about his deceased parents. KK's spouse reported that he frequently called his children by the wrong names, which has been a cause of increased anxiety and concern for the family. About 3 weeks ago, KK's wife went to the store for about an hour and upon her return the door of the house was open and the water in the kitchen sink was running. KK was found wandering in the streets and was brought back by the police. KK did not remember this incident. The wife reported that he seemed to have poor impulse control at times when he was confused and frustrated, as he would yell and swing his arms. She has been feeling unsafe for him and for herself taking care of him at home, as he has been requiring constant supervision. During the interview the client was calm, verbally responsive and cooperative, behaviorally in control despite his difficulty answering various questions and often delayed in his responses.

C. *Past Psychiatric History*

KK denied any prior psychiatric illness or related treatment, including outpatient or inpatient hospitalizations, which was confirmed by his wife.

D. *Substance Use History*

KK denies any substance use. He reports having a glass of wine with his dinner two or three times a week for the last 20 years. He denies any history of smoking or any use of illegal drugs. KK's wife confirmed the given information.

E. *Social and Developmental History*

1. *Education*: Graduated with a bachelor's degree, majoring in engineering science.
2. *Family Relationships, Social Network, and Abuse History*: The client is domiciled, married for 45 years, has three children and five grandchildren. The children and grandchildren visit periodically, and he always enjoys being with all his family, especially during the holidays. However, over the last year, as his forgetfulness has gotten worse, he has become increasingly irritated when the house is full with his children, their spouses, and the grandchildren. The client's wife reported that he was a good father to the children and had been very welcoming toward the grandchildren when he was well.

    Socially, he had many social and close friends until his forgetfulness began to affect his functions, including driving, going out to various events, and talking on the phone. At this point, he is no longer able to stay connected with people outside of his immediate family. No known history of physical, psychological, or sexual abuse reported.

3. *Employment Record and/or Military History*: Worked as an engineer for the Navy for over 30 years and retired 10 years ago.
4. *Legal Record*: No legal issues reported.
5. *Religious Background*: Practicing Anglican.

F. *Family Psychiatric History*

Both parents are deceased. There is no known AD on either the client's maternal or paternal side. Also, no known family history of mental illness reported.

G. *Review of Systems*

1. Vital signs: BP: 120/80; HR: 70; RR: 20; Temp: 98 F; Ht: 5'10"; Wt: 200 lbs.
2. Review of systems showed no significant observable overall physical abnormalities; alert and oriented to name and place, but not to date and time.
   - No peripheral edema.
   - Wearing reading glasses, no hearing aid required.
   - No tinnitus, vertigo.
   - No infection at present time reported.
   - No heart or pulmonary problems reported.
   - High blood pressure under control with amlodipine 5 mg daily.
   - Hypercholesterolemia under control with simvastatin 20 mg po daily.
3. Allergies: No known allergies reported.
4. Had a physical examination with his PCP a week ago and was reported to be "physically healthy" (will obtain a copy of the physical examination).

H. *Mental Status Examination*

1. *Appearance and Behavior*: The client appeared to be the stated age. He was noted to stare blankly at times during the interview, but responded to questions appropriately with short sentences. His hygiene was fair, adequately dressed for the weather.
2. *Mood*: Euthymic.
3. *Affect*: Constricted and mood congruent.
4. *Thought Content and Process*: Speech rate and volume were clear but delayed response to some questions noted and required repeating of some questions before answering. He presented no evidence of loose associations, tangential thoughts, or thought blocking.
5. *Perceptual Disturbances*: The client denied delusions or paranoia, but his wife reported that at times he became suspicious and accusatory toward his children, claiming that they were taking advantage of him. Denied auditory/visual/tactile hallucinations.
6. *Sensorium, Cognitive, and Intellectual Functioning*: The client is oriented × 2. He is unable to accurately state the current date and time. His insight and judgment were impaired, as the illness has progressed.

I. *Diagnosis and Treatment Plan*

1. **DSM-5 Diagnosis:** Possible major NCD due to AD without serious behavioral disturbance.
2. **Rationale for Diagnostic Impression:** In this section, a table format is used to present the information (see Table 2.27). This is different from the format used for the previous disorders to introduce the APMHN to other ways of organizing information when determining the diagnosis.

Diagnostic Assessment and Screening Inventories

1. The MMSE completed, the client scored 10 out of a maximum 30 points, which indicates that he has moderate cognitive impairment. MMSE is not a diagnostic instrument but measures the degree of cognitive impairment. The scores are generally grouped as follows:
   - 25–30 points: Normal cognition.
   - 21–24 points: Mild cognitive impairment.
   - 10–20 points: Moderate cognitive impairment.
   - 9 points or lower: Severe cognitive impairment.
2. The Short Portable Mental Status Questionnaire (SPMSQ) contains ten questions to assess organic brain deficit in elderly clients. KK scored seven errors out of ten questions, indicating moderate cognitive impairment. The scores are generally grouped as follows:
   - 0–2 errors: Normal mental functioning.
   - 3–4 errors: Mild cognitive impairment.
   - 5–7 errors: Moderate cognitive impairment.
   - 8 or more errors: Severe cognitive impairment.

   Other instruments are also available to measure the cognitive, visuospatial, and functional status of a person who may have suspected NCDs. For example:
3. The Clock Drawing Test is a simple tool that is usually used to determine the client's visuospatial disorganization of time.
4. The scales of functional assessment of activities of daily living (ADL) are instruments used to evaluate an individual's functional state in a systematic, individualized way. Three scales are currently available: (1) basic activities of daily living (BADL); (2) instrumental activities of daily living (IADL); and (3) advanced activities of daily living (AADL).

Final diagnosis is confirmed as possible major NCD due to AD without serious behavioral disturbance.

3. *Treatment Plan*
   - Collaborative approach with the PCP and a geriatric specialist for further evaluation, including medications and diagnostic markers for AD:

Table 2.27 Rationale for NCD due to AD Diagnostic Criteria Matching with the Client's Symptoms

Major Neurocognitive Disorder	The Client's Symptoms
A.	Evidence of significant cognitive decline from a previous level of performance in one or more cognitive domains based on A1 and A2:	
A1.	Concern of the individual, a knowledgeable informant, or the clinician that there has been a significant decline in cognitive function; and	A1. The client's wife reported that the client's memory and independent functions have deteriorated significantly over the last year, and is concerned about his safety and inability to care for himself without full supervision.
A2.	A substantial impairment in cognitive performance, preferably documented by standardized neuropsychological testing or, in its absence, another quantified clinical assessment.	A2. During the initial psychiatric evaluation, it was confirmed that the client showed a substantial impairment in his cognitive performance, based on the personal interview evaluation as well as an MMSE score of 10.
B.	The cognitive deficits interfere with independence in everyday activities (i.e., at a minimum, requiring assistance with complex instrumental activities of daily living, such as paying bills or managing medications).	B. The client's cognitive impairment led his wife to believe that it may not be safe to leave him alone, as evidenced by his wandering behavior, his inability to perform a simple task, such as making a phone call or following a simple direction, and his requiring supervision to prevent any exposure to risk, such as being lost outside of the house.
C.	The cognitive deficits do not occur exclusively in the context of delirium.	C. No evidence of delirium noted during the evaluation.
D.	The cognitive deficits are not better explained by a mental disorder (e.g., major depressive disorder, schizophrenia).	D. No evidence of mental disorders detected, including depression, psychosis, bipolar disorders.

(Continued)

Table 2.27 (Continued)

Probable *vs.* Possible *Major Neurocognitive Disorder due to AD*	The Client's *Symptom Presentation*
Probable AD is diagnosed if either of the following is present; otherwise, possible AD should be diagnosed:	Possible AD is diagnosed until a full neurological evaluation to rule out other NCDs or systematic disease or condition likely contributing to cognitive decline.
1. Evidence of a causative AD genetic mutation from family history or genetic testing. 2. All three of the following are present:	1. No evidence of family history or genetic testing (no evidence of family history). 2. All three of the following are present for this client:
a. Clear evidence of decline in memory and learning, and at least one other cognitive domain (based on detailed history or serial neuropsychological testing).	a. Clear evidence of decline in memory and learning; based on detailed history, the client met impairment in cognitive domain. Major complex attention deficits manifested by difficulty in environments with multiple stimuli (agitated during family gatherings), holding new information, unable to perform mental calculation ("don't remember where I am at times, and I find it difficult to remember if I have paid my bills"), all thinking takes longer than usual (delayed responses during the interview).
b. Steadily progressive, gradual decline in cognition, without extended plateaus.	b. Steadily progressive, gradual decline in cognition without extended plateaus are evidenced by the gradual deterioration of the client's memory, affecting his cognitive functioning, social and familiar interactions, and ability to care for himse f.
c. No evidence of mixed etiology (i.e., absence of other neurogenerative or cerebrovascular disease, or another neurological, mental, or systematic disease or condition likely contributing to cognitive decline).	c. There is no mixed etiology of other medical or mental conditions reported; however, a full neurological evaluation o rule out other NCDs or systematic disease is required to make a probable AD diagnosis.

- CT or MRI to evaluate diffuse cortical atrophy, enlarged ventricle, and decreased brain acetylcholine metabolism.
- Amyloid-based diagnostic test, such as amyloid imaging on brain positron emission tomography scans.
- Cerebrospinal fluid test to determine any reduced levels of amyloid beta-42.
- Genetic testing, if requested by the client and family, for a mutation in one of the known causative AD genes: amyloid precursor protein, presenilin 1, or presenilin 2. Genetic testing for such mutations is available, at least for PSEN1.

- Referral to social services to coordinate issues relating to patient safety, finances, and legal planning.
- Recommend that the family seek additional supports and education from the local Alzheimer's Association chapter.

Section 10: Personality Disorders

A personality disorder is an enduring pattern of inner experience and external behavior characterized by inflexible and unhealthy patterns of thinking, feeling, and behaving. These experiences and behaviors often deviate markedly from the expectations of the individual's culture, and can lead to unhappiness and impairment. They manifest in at least two of the following four areas: cognition, affectivity, interpersonal function, and impulse control. Also, when personality traits are rigid and maladaptive, an individual experiences functional impairment or subjective stress. The onset of personality disorders usually starts in adolescence or early adulthood. Personality disorders include ten distinctively specified disorders, which are explained in more detail in Table 2.28: (1) paranoid, (2) schizoid, (3) schizotypal, (4) histrionic, (5) narcissistic, (6) antisocial, (7) borderline, (8) avoidant, (9) dependent, and (10) obsessive-compulsive (Sadock et al., 2019). A national epidemiological survey of general population data suggests a prevalence of paranoid personality disorder of 4.4%, schizoid personality disorder of 3.1%, schizotypal personality disorder of 3.9%, and dependent personality disorder of 0.6% (APA, 2013). The prevalence of other personality disorders in the general population are as follows: antisocial personality disorder is 3% in men and 1% in women; borderline personality disorder is about 2%, more common in women than in men; histrionic personality disorder is 2–3%; narcissistic personality disorder is less than 1%; obsessive-compulsive personality disorder is 1%; avoidance personality disorder is 0.05–1% (Sadock et al., 2019).

The DSM-5 (APA, 2013) groups personality disorders into three clusters and one category of personality disorder traits:

1. **Cluster A.** *The odd and eccentric cluster*, which consists of paranoid, schizoid, and schizotypal personality disorders. These disorders are characterized by the use of fantasy and projection, associated with a tendency toward psychotic thinking. Cognitive disorganization may be common.

Table 2.28 General Characteristics of Specific Personality Disorders

Personality Disorder	*Essential Diagnostic Features*
Paranoid	Pervasive distrust and suspiciousness of others, often interpreting their motives as malevolent and, as a result, becoming hostile, irritable, hypersensitive, envious, or angry
Schizoid	Pervasive pattern of detachment from social relations; an isolated lifestyle and lack of interest in social interaction, with a restricted range of expression of emotions in interpersonal settings
Schizotypal	Pervasive pattern of social and interpersonal deficits marked by acute discomfort with, and reduced capacity for, close relationships, as well as by cognitive or perceptual distortions and behavioral eccentricities
Histrionic	Pervasive and emotionally excessive attention-seeking behaviors
Narcissistic	Pervasive patterns of grandiosity, need for admiration, and lack of empathy
Antisocial	Pervasive patterns of disregard for, and violation of, the rights of others, also deceitful and manipulative; this pattern is also referred to as psychopathy or sociopathy
Borderline	Pervasive pattern of instability of interpersonal relationships, self-image, affects, and marked impulsivity
Avoidant	Pervasive pattern of social inhibition, feelings of inadequacy, and hypersensitivity to negative evaluation
Dependent	Pervasive and excessive need to be taken care of that leads to submissive and clinging behavior and fears of separation
Obsessive-compulsive	Preoccupation with orderliness, perfectionism, and mental and interpersonal control, at the expense of flexibility, openness, and efficiency

Source: Adapted from DSM-5, APA (2013).

2. **Cluster B.** *The dramatic, emotional, and erratic cluster*, which consists of histrionic, narcissistic, antisocial, and borderline personality disorders. These disorders are characterized by symptoms of dissociation, denial, splitting, and acting out. Mood disorders may be common.

3. **Cluster C.** *The anxious or fearful cluster*, which consists of avoidant, dependent, and obsessive-compulsive personality disorders. These disorders are characterized by the use of isolation, passive aggressiveness, and hypochondriasis.

4. **Personality disorder traits** refers to individuals who frequently exhibit traits that are not limited to a single personality disorder. When personality traits are rigid and maladaptive, and produce functional impairment or subjective distress, *general personality disorder* may be diagnosed.

In this section, borderline personality disorder is chosen as an example to address the mental status assessment and diagnostic evaluation of personality disorders, as it represents the classic condition in this group of disorders.

The prevalence of borderline personality disorder is approximately 2% in the general population, predominantly (75%) in females. Physical and sexual abuse, neglect, hostile conflict, and early parental loss are common in the childhood histories of individuals with this disorder. Of clients with borderline personality disorders, 90% have one other psychiatric diagnosis, and 40% have two (Sadock et al., 2019). Common psychiatric comorbidities are depressive and bipolar disorders, substance use disorders, eating disorders (notably bulimia nervosa), PTSD, and attention-deficit/hyperactivity disorder (APA, 2013). Clients with borderline personality disorder exhibit extraordinarily unstable mood, affect, behavior, object relations, and self-image. They are marked by pervasive and excessive instability in interpersonal relationships, significant mood swings, impulsive behavior with regard to money and sex, and often engage in substance abuse, reckless driving, or binge eating. Self-destructive, self-mutilating, and suicide gestures, threats, or attempts occur frequently. They tend to have micro-psychotic episodes, often with paranoia and transient dissociative symptoms. They also suffer from identity problems, as well as from feelings of emptiness and boredom, and always appear to be in a state of crisis (Sadock et al., 2019).

Diagnostic Criteria

DSM-5 Borderline Personality Disorder Criteria Modified

A. **Signs and Symptoms:** Pervasive pattern of instability in interpersonal relationships, self-image, and affects, marked impulsivity, beginning by early adulthood and present in a variety of contexts, as indicated by five (or more) of the following symptom criteria:
1. Recurrent suicidal behavior, gestures, or threats, or self-mutilating behavior.
2. Frantic efforts to avoid real or imagined abandonment.
3. Impulsivity in at least two areas that are potentially self-damaging (e.g., spending, sex, substance abuse, reckless driving, binge eating).
4. A pattern of unstable and intense interpersonal relationships, characterized by alternations between extremes of idealization and devaluation.
5. Identity disturbance; markedly and persistently unstable self-image or sense of self.
6. Affective instability due to a marked reactivity of mood (e.g., intense episodic dysphoria, irritability, or anxiety, usually lasting a few hours or, rarely, more than a few days).
7. Chronic feelings of emptiness.
8. Inappropriate, intense anger or difficulty controlling anger (e.g., frequent displays of temper, constant anger, recurrent physical fights).
9. Transient, stress-related paranoid ideation or severe dissociative symptoms.
B. **Differential Diagnosis:** Borderline personality disorder often co-occurs with depressive disorder or bipolar disorder; when criteria for both are met, both may be diagnosed.

Interviewing Techniques in Assessment of
Borderline Personality Disorder

The following are samples of diagnostic interview questions designed to help the APMHN to elicit the symptoms of borderline personality disorder during the initial psychiatric evaluation of a client. Following the above DSM-5 diagnostic criteria of borderline personality disorder, sample interview questions are created with a rationale to evaluate each symptom criteria.

Criterion 1: Recurrent suicidal behavior, gestures, or threats, or self-mutilating behavior
   Questions:

   1. Have you had thoughts of wanting to kill yourself? If you have, have you acted on them?

(This is an open-ended question to explore the client's suicidal ideation, intention, plan, and attempt(s). There is a myth that asking the client directly about suicidal ideation might give them the idea to kill themselves. To the contrary, open discussion of suicide could convey that suicidal ideation is no longer a sin to be hidden, but rather a problem to be solved and that help may be only a spoken word away [Shea, 1998a].*)*

   2. Have you ever mutilated yourself, such as cutting your wrists, burning yourself with cigarette butts, or any other ways of hurting yourself?

(Clients with borderline personality disorder tend to cut or burn themselves, and it's common that they report no pain. Self-mutilation seems to serve as a release for intense feelings of rage, often preceded by an argument or a broken relationship.)

Criterion 2: Frantic efforts to avoid real or imagined abandonment
   Question: Are you often afraid that others may leave you or abandon you, so you try to make every effort to stop them from leaving you (even when it's not real)?

Criterion 3: Impulsivity in at least two areas that are potentially self-damaging (e.g., spending, sex, substance abuse, reckless driving, binge eating)
   Question: Have you found yourself doing one or more of the following: driving recklessly, engaging in unsafe sex, abusing alcohol or drugs, binge eating, gambling, or spending money recklessly?
   (These clients frequently view life as boring, and coupled with their intense feelings of self-loathing, they ceaselessly seek stimulation, using drugs, engaging in unsafe sex, and binge eating to satisfy their feelings of emptiness.)

Criterion 4: A pattern of unstable and intense interpersonal relationships characterized by alternating between extremes of idealization and devaluation

Question: When you meet people, do you find yourself very comfortable sharing the most intimate details with them? And do you then feel that these same people don't care and are not there enough for you? For example, have you experienced that most of your romantic relationships have been very intense, but not very stable?

Criterion 5: Identity disturbance; markedly and persistently unstable self-image or sense of self

Question: Do you often experience a sudden shift in the way you look at yourself and your life, and do you completely change your goals, values, and career focus?

Criterion 6: Affective instability due to a marked reactivity of mood (e.g., intense episodic dysphoria, irritability, or anxiety, usually lasting a few hours or, rarely, more than a few days)

Question: Do you find yourself at times highly sensitive and overly reactive to things happening in your life, and your mood becoming extremely irritable, anxious, or depressed for a short time?

Criterion 7: Chronic feelings of emptiness

Question: Do you often feel emptiness inside you unless you are around other people?

(*These clients often experience life with no sense of inner self other than hollowness. Therefore, they tend to depend on others to give meaning to life. Consequently, they intensely dislike being alone and develop dependency on others, as well as fear of abandonment.*)

Criterion 8: Inappropriate, intense anger or difficulty controlling anger (e.g., frequent displays of temper, constant anger, recurrent physical fights)

Question: Do you sometimes feel extremely angry and bitter for no apparent reason, and have a hard time controlling these feelings, engaging in verbal or physical altercations, or violence?

Criterion 9: Transient, stress-related paranoid ideation or severe dissociative symptoms

Question: When you are stressed out, especially if you feel abandoned or betrayed by someone, have you found yourself being very paranoid, or feeling "spaced out" or having "out-of-body" experiences?

The following is a sample case exemplar of the initial psychiatric evaluation, including the rationale of how the diagnosis of borderline personality disorder is determined, and the proposed preliminary treatment plan. As indicated earlier, a client with borderline personality disorder presents a high likelihood of comorbid psychiatric disorder(s); therefore, it is essential for the APMHN to be mindful of evaluating the client while conducting the initial interview.

Case Exemplar

The client's initials are AF.

Initial Psychiatric Evaluation

A. *Identification, Chief Complaint, and Reason for Referral*

AF is a 22-year-old Hispanic-American male, referred to the outpatient mental health clinic from the local hospital, where he stayed overnight for observation following an attempt to cut himself with a pocket knife. His chief complaint was, "I feel like crap." The client was accompanied by his mother.

B. *History of Present Illness*

Two days ago, AF's brother took him to the local hospital, where he was admitted overnight and then discharged with a referral to the mental health clinic. The client's family reported that the brother found him cutting himself with a pocket knife and called 911. As per the client, he broke up with his girlfriend about 2 months ago, and just found out that she was pregnant with another man's baby. AF became furious, even though he was no longer in a relationship with her, and felt the urge to cut himself. He reported a prior cutting incident, and also an attempt to commit suicide once in the past by overdosing on pills.

As per the hospital discharge summary, the left wrist cuts made by the client at the time of the hospital admission were superficial and did not require any suturing. However, he was kept overnight for observation, and then discharged to the outpatient mental health clinic, as he denied suicidal ideation, intent, or plans. The client's mother reported that AF got easily upset and irritable, and was unhappy with his life. He often became argumentative with the mother and the brother, losing his temper and punching the walls and doors, usually for about 3–4 hours. The mother also reported that each time he threw a temper tantrum, he made threats of killing himself, which made both the mother and brother concerned about him. During the interview, the client was cooperative, responded appropriately to questions, and denied feeling depressed. However, AF claimed that ever since he was an adolescent, he has often felt empty inside, accompanied by loneliness. When asked about his recent hospitalization, he claimed that he terminated the relationship with his ex-girlfriend, but when he found out recently that she was pregnant by another man, he had intense feelings of betrayal and rage, followed by feeling numb and becoming totally spaced out. The next thing he did was try to cut his wrist, and he did not even feel any pain while doing it. He claimed that he did not intend to kill himself at the time, and denied any suicidal ideation/intent/plan. He also denied any signs of psychosis, including hallucinations, delusions, paranoia, or any other thought disorders. He is oriented to date, time and place, and his cognitive functions are fully intact.

C. *Past Psychiatric History*

AF was diagnosed with bipolar disorder when he was 17 years old and treated with Depakote 250 mg twice a day, but he claimed that the medication did not help his mood swings and angry outbursts, so he stopped taking it and did not follow up with the treatment. AF had a history of two previous hospitalizations. One was in 2015, when he took an overdose, ingesting 10 pills of 250 mg Depakote following a verbal altercation with his mother and brother. He was hospitalized for 4 days and was discharged with the recommendation to follow up with outpatient treatment, but he did not. The second hospitalization was 2 months ago, when he was found cutting his left wrist with a pocket knife following the break-up with his girlfriend. He was evaluated at the comprehensive psychiatric emergency program (CPEP), and the injury from the cut was found to be superficial, non-bleeding, and didn't need suturing. He was discharged from the CPEP with the assessment that he did not require inpatient treatment, and was referred to the outpatient mental health clinic, but did not follow up.

D. *Substance Use History*

AF denied any substance use, including alcohol, cannabis, cocaine, heroin, opiates, or benzodiazepines. However, he reported smoking six cigarettes per day and said he has no intention of quitting.

E. *Social and Developmental History*

1. *Education*: AF completed high school and planned to go to college, but was not sure what he wanted to study.
2. *Family Relationships, Social Network, and Abuse History*: AF lives with his mother and his older brother in a three-bedroom apartment. He often gets into arguments with them; however, he believes that they are trying to help him and he hopes to have a decent relationship with them. AF reported that his father left the family when he was about 9 years old, and remembered that his father was very strict when he was a child. AF's mother reported that his father was physically abusive toward AF during his childhood, but AF was reluctant to talk about his relationship with the father; he blamed himself for his father leaving him and his family because his father was angry at him since AF was not a good son. AF is currently not in any intimate relationship, but reported that each of his relationships has lasted less than a year and each time he is the one who terminates it, saying "Everyone leaves me eventually anyway." He further elaborated that most of his relationships have been very chaotic, with ups and downs like a roller-coaster. AF's social activities are limited to his cousins, with whom he spends most of his time.
3. *Employment Record and/or Military History*: AF has a history of working at different places for a short period of time. He currently works 10–15 hours per week at a moving company. He does freelance writing, but is not clear about the details of his work. He doesn't have a military history.

4. *Legal Record*: AF denied having a history of legal issues.
5. *Religious Background*: AF identifies as Roman Catholic, but is not religious.

F. **Family History of Psychiatric Illnesses**

AF's father was an alcoholic, but, other than that, AF denied having a history of mental illness in the family.

G. **Medical History and Review of Systems**

1. Review of systems: No visible abnormality noted other than three superficial marks of redness on his left wrist from the attempt to cut.
2. AF's medical record from the hospital where he was discharged revealed no significant physical illness and no medications prescribed.
3. No known allergies reported.

H. **Mental Status Examination**

1. *Appearance and Behavior*: The client appeared to be the stated age and cleanly shaven, casually dressed in T-shirt and blue jeans. He presented with calm, cooperative behaviors and was easily engaged in the interview, with good eye contact.
2. *Mood*: Euthymic.
3. *Affect*: Mood congruent.
4. *Thought Content and Process*: Speech was within a normal range with rate, rhythm, and volume. Thought process was linear, goal oriented, and coherent, with no evidence of delusion or any other thought disorders present.
5. *Perceptual Disturbances*: Thought contents were nonpsychotic; he denied having any auditory/visual hallucinations, and denied having any suicidal/homicidal ideations, plans, or intentions. The client claimed that his self-mutilation gesture was not a suicidal attempt, but rather was an impulsive reaction to life stressors.
6. *Sensorium, Cognitive, and Intellectual Functioning*: Alert and oriented to time, place, and person. No evidence of cognitive impairment, and average intellectual functioning noted.

I. **Diagnosis and Treatment Plan**

1. **DSM-5 Diagnosis**: Borderline personality disorder.
2. **Rationale for Diagnostic Criteria**: According to the DSM-5 (APA, 2013), the following criteria must be present to diagnose borderline personality disorder: *pervasive* pattern of instability in interpersonal relationships, self-image, and affects, marked impulsivity, beginning by early adulthood and present in a variety of contexts, as indicated by five (or more) of the nine symptom criteria. The client meets those criteria, as indicated by the bold symptom categories:
   1. **Recurrent suicidal behavior, gestures, or threats, or self-mutilating behavior.** AF has made multiple threats of committing suicide, with one attempt by medication overdose, and has had two incidents of self-mutilation by cutting his wrist.

2. *Frantic efforts to avoid real or imagined abandonment.* All of AF's intimate relationships have lasted less than a year and each time he was the one who terminated the relationship, saying "Everyone leaves me eventually anyway."

3. Impulsivity in at least two areas that are potentially self-damaging (e.g., spending, sex, substance abuse, reckless driving, binge eating).

4. *A pattern of unstable and intense interpersonal relationships, characterized by* alternating between extremes of idealization and devaluation. Most of AF's intimate relationships have been very chaotic, with ups and downs like a roller-coaster.

5. *Identity disturbance; markedly and persistently unstable self-image or sense of self.* AF was reluctant to talk about his relationship with the father and blamed himself for his father leaving him and his family because his father was angry at him since he was "not a good son."

6. *Affective instability due to a marked reactivity of mood (e.g., intense episodic dysphoria, irritability, or anxiety, usually lasting a few hours or, rarely, more than a few days).* AF's mother reported that AF became easily upset and irritable, and was unhappy with his life.

7. *Chronic feeling of emptiness.* AF reported feelings of emptiness, accompanied by loneliness, since he was an adolescent.

8. *Inappropriate, intense anger or difficulty controlling anger.* He often became angry and argumentative with the mother and the brother, followed by losing his temper and eventually punching the walls and doors, which usually lasted for 3–4 hours.

9. *Transient, stress-related paranoid ideation or severe dissociative symptoms.* When AF got angry about his ex-girlfriend, he experienced intense feelings of betrayal, followed by numbness and being totally spaced out.

The client's final diagnosis is confirmed as borderline personality disorder, evidenced by meeting eight of the borderline personality disorder symptom criteria (requirement is the presence of five [or more] of the symptom criteria).

3. *Treatment Plan*:

- There is proven evidence that dialectical behavior therapy (DBT) is one of the most effective forms of psychotherapy for borderline personality disorder (Choi-Kain et al., 2017). Therefore, AF could be referred to a DBT-trained therapist.
- AF was diagnosed with bipolar disorder when he was 17 years old and is currently not being treated for it. Therefore, a thorough investigation of bipolar disorder as a potential comorbid psychiatric disorder should be done.
- A multimodal approach involving family psychoeducation, and family systems or dynamic intervention where possible, in combination with medications and individual psychotherapy, is recommended.

References

American Psychiatric Association (APA). (2013). *Diagnostic and statistical manual of mental disorders (DSM-5)* (5th ed., text rev.). Author.

American Psychiatric Association (APA). (2016). *Practice guidelines for the psychiatric evaluation of adults* (3rd ed.). American Psychiatric Association. https://doi.org/10 .1176/appi.pn.2015.8a5

Barry, P. (2005). Interpersonal psychotherapy. In K. Wheeler (Ed.), *Psychotherapy for the advanced practice nurse* (pp. 203–221). Mosby Elsevier.

Choi-Kain, L. W., Finch, E. F., Masland, S. R., Jenkins, J. A., & Unruh, B. T. (2017). What works in the treatment of borderline personality disorder. *Current Behavioral Neuroscience Reports, 4*(1), 21–30. https://doi.org/10.1007/s40473-017-0103-z

Citrome, L. (2011). Neurochemical models of schizophrenia: Transcending dopamine. *Current Psychiatry (Supplement), 10*(9), S10–S14.

De Vries, Y., Roest, A., Bos, E., Burgerhof, J., Van Loo, H., & De Jonge, P. (2019). Predicting antidepressant response by monitoring early improvement of individual symptoms of depression: Individual patient data meta-analysis. *British Journal of Psychiatry, 214*(1), 4–10. https://doi.org/10.1192/bjp.2018.122

Frank, G., Shott, M. E., & DeGuzman, M. C. (2019). The neurobiology of eating disorders. *Child and Adolescent Psychiatric Clinics of North America, 28*(4), 629–640. https:// doi10.1016/j.chc.2019.05.007. www.researchgate.net/publication/334234590

Furuta, M., Horsch, A., Ng, E. S. W., Bick, D., Spain, D., & Sin, J. (2018). Effectiveness of trauma-focused psychological therapies for treating post-traumatic stress disorder symptoms in women following childbirth: A systematic review and meta-analysis. *Frontiers in Psychiatry, 9*(591), 1–17. ISSN 1664-6640. https://doi.org/10.3389/fpsyt .2018.00591

Guerrera, C. S., Furneri, G., Grasso, M., Caruso, G., Castellano, S., Drago, F., Di-Nuovo, S., & Caraci, F. (2020). Antidepressant drugs and physical activity: A possible synergism in the treatment of major depression? *Frontiers in Psychology, 11*(857), 1–9. https://doi .org/10.3389/fpsyg.2020.00857

Hay, P., Chinn, D., Forbes, D., Madden, S., Newton, R., Sugenor, L., Touyz, S., & Ward, W. (2014). Royal Australian and New Zealand College of Psychiatrist clinical practice guidelines for the treatment of eating disorders. *Australian New Zealand Journal of Psychiatry, 48*, 977–1008.

Heerema, E. (2019). Talking to a loved one who has dementia: Effective communication strategies in Alzheimer's. *Verywell Health.* www.verywellhealth.com/how-to-talk-to -someone-with-dementia-97963

Information for Practice. (2012, December 8). Lifetime prevalence of DSM-IV/WMH-CIDI disorders by sex and cohort. https://ifp.nyu.edu/2012/infographics/lifetime -prevalence-of-dsm-ivwmh-cidi-disorders-by-sex-and-cohort-n9282/

Jaggar, M., Fanibunda, S. E., Ghosh, S., Duman, R. S., & Vaidya, V. A. (2019). Chapter: The neurotrophic hypothesis of depression revisited: New insights and therapeutic implications. *Neurobiology of Depression, 367*, 43–62. https://doi:10.1016/ B978-0-12-813333-0.00006-8

Kadriu, B., Musazzi, L., Henter, I. D., Graves, M., Popoli, M., &Zarate Jr, C. A. (2019). Glutamatergic neurotransmission: Pathway to developing novel rapid-acting antidepressant treatments. *International Journal of Neuropsychopharmacology, 22*, 119–135.

Kaltenboeck, A., & Harmer, C. (2018). The neuroscience of depressive disorders: A brief review of the past and some considerations about the future. *Brain and Neuroscience Advances, 2*, 1–6. https://doi.org/10.1177/2398212818799269

Kessler, R. C., & Bromet, E. J. (2013). The epidemiology of depression across cultures. *Annual Review of Public Health, 34,* 119–138. https://doi:10.1146/annurev-publhealth-031912-114409

Lipari, R. N., & Van Horn, S. L. (2017, June 29). *Trends in substance use disorders among adults aged 18 or older.* The CBHSQ Report. Center for Behavioral Health Statistics and Quality, Substance Abuse and Mental Health Services Administration.

McCance, K., & Huether, S. (2018). *Pathophysiology: The biologic basis for disease in adults and children* (8th ed.). Mosby Publisher. ISBN 9780323583473/0323583474

Nakao, T., Okada, K., & Kanba, S. (2014). Neurobiological model of obsessive–compulsive disorder: Evidence from recent neuropsychological and neuroimaging findings. *Psychiatry and Clinical Neurosciences, 68*(8), 587–605.

National Institutes of Alcohol Abuse and Alcoholism (NIAAA) (2021). Alcohol facts and statistics. www.niaaa.nih.gov/publications/brochures-and-fact-sheets/alcohol-facts-and-statistics

National Institutes of Health (NIH) (2015, November 18). Newsletter: 10 percent of US adults have drug use disorder at some point in their lives. www.nih.gov/news-events/news-releases/10-percent-us-adults-have-drug-use-disorder-some-point-their-lives

National Institutes of Health: National Institute on Alcohol Abuse and Alcoholism (NIH–NIAAA) (2020, December). Understanding alcohol use disorder. www.niaaa.nih.gov/sites/default/files/publications/Alcohol_Use_Disorder.pdf

Phillips, M. S., & Kupfer, D. J. (2013). Bipolar disorder diagnosis: Challenges and future directions. *Lancet, 381*(9878), 1663–1671.

Pietrabissa, G., Manzoni, G. M., Gibson, P. J., Boardman, D. V., Gori, A., & Castelnuovo, G. (2016). Brief strategic therapy for obsessive compulsive disorder: A clinical and research protocol of a one-group observational study. *British Medical Journal, 6*(3), e009118. https://doi:10.1136/bmjopen-2015009118

Psych Scene Hub. (n.d.). Schizophrenia: Diagnostic interview. https://psychscenehub.com/psychpedia/schizophrenia-diagnostic-interview/

Sadock, B., & Sadock, V. (2010). *Kaplan & Sadock's Pocket handbook of clinical psychiatry* (5th ed.). Wolters Kluwer/Lippincott Williams & Wilkins.

Sadock, B., Ahmad, S., & Sadock, V. (2019). *Kaplan & Sadock's pocket handbook of clinical psychiatry* (6th ed.). Wolters Kluwer.

Saxena, S., Brody, A. L., Maidment, K. M., Dunkin, J. J., Colgan, M., Alborzian, S., Phelps, M. E., & Baxter, Jr., L. R. (1998). Localized orbitofrontal and subcortical metabolic changes and predictors of response to paroxetine treatment in obsessive compulsive disorder. *Neuropsychopharmacology, 21*(6), 683–693.

Shea, S. C. (1998). *Psychiatric interviewing: The art of understanding* (2nd ed.). W.B. Saunders. ISBN-13: 978-0721670119

Spitzer, R. L., Kroenke, K., Williams, J. B., & Löwe, B. (2006). A brief measure for assessing generalized anxiety disorder: The GAD-7. *Archives of General Internal Medicine, 166*(10), 1092–1097. https://doi:10.1001/archinte.166.10.1092

Stahl, S. M. (2013). *Essential psychopharmacology: Neuroscientific bases and practical applications* (4th ed.). Cambridge University Press.

Tracy, N. (2012). Effects of bipolar disorder. HealthyPlace. www.healthyplace.com/bipolar-disorder/bipolar-information/effects-of-bipolar-disorder

Trygstad, L. N., Buccheri, R. K., Buffum, M. D., Dau-shen, J., & Dowling, G. A. (2015). Auditory hallucinations interview guide: Promoting recovery with an interactive assessment tool. *Journal of Psychosocial Nursing and Mental Health Services, 53*(1), 20–28. https://doi.org/10.3928/02793695-20141203-01

Van der Kolk, B. (2006). Clinical implications of neuroscience research in PTSD. *Annals of New York Academy of Sciences, 1071*(1), 277–293.

Victoria Department of Hospital & Health Services (DHHS); Victoria's Hub for Health Services & Business. (2021). Differential diagnosis: Depression, delirium and dementia.   www2.health.vic.gov.au/hospitals-and-health-services/patient-care/older -people/cognition/diff-diagnosis

Villarroel, M. A., & Terlizzi, E. P. (2020, September). Symptoms of depression among adults: United States, 2019. NCHS Data Brief, no 379. National Center for Health Statistics. www.cdc.gov/nchs/products/index.htm

Yatham, L. N., Kennedy, S. H., Parikh, S. V., Schaffer, A., Bond, D. J., Frey, B. N., Sharma, V., Goldstein, B. I., Rej, S., Beaulieu, S., Alda, M., MacQueen, G., Milev, R. V., Ravindran, A., O'Donovan, C., McIntosh, D., Lam, R. W., Vazquez, G., Kapczinski, F., … Berk, M. (2018). Canadian Network for Mood and Anxiety Treatments (CANMAT) and International Society for Bipolar Disorders (ISBD) 2018 guidelines for the management of patients with bipolar disorder. *Bipolar Disorders, 20*(2), 97–170. https://doi.org/10.1111/bdi.12609

Zisook, S. (2005). Death, dying, and bereavement. In B. J. Sadock & V. A. Sadock (Eds.), *Comprehensive textbook of psychiatry* (8th ed.) (pp. 2367–2393). Lippincott, Williams & Wilkins.

3 Practice Guidelines for the Assessment of Risk for Violent Behaviors during the Psychiatric Evaluation

Violence is defined as the intentional threat or actual use of physical force or power against oneself, a group, or a community that results in or has a high likelihood of resulting in injury, death, psychological harm, maldevelopment, and/or deprivation. There are two types of violence: (1) self-directed violence, such as suicide; and (2) other-directed violence, such as aggressive behaviors, including physical aggression or homicide. More than 1.3 million people worldwide die each year as a result of violence in all its forms, accounting for 2.5% of global mortality (World Health Organization [WHO], 2014).

The WHO (2019) reported that suicide is a global phenomenon that can occur throughout the lifespan. Approximately 800,000 people worldwide die by suicide each year, which is one person every 40 seconds. As of 2016, suicide accounted for 1.4% of all deaths worldwide, making it the 18th leading cause of death; 79% occurred in low- and middle-income countries. Furthermore, there are indications that for each adult who dies by suicide, more than 20 others may have attempted it (WHO, 2019). In the United States, approximately 40,000 people commit suicide each year, a rate of 12.5 deaths per 100,000 annually, and approximately 250,000 people attempt suicide each year (Sadock et al., 2019).

Homicide is also a global phenomenon. As of 2012, the latest year for which figures are available, an estimated 475,000 deaths occurred worldwide as a result of homicide. Of these, 60% were males aged 15–44 years, making homicide the third leading cause of death for males in this age group; overall, 82% of homicide deaths were males (6.7 per 100,000 population) (WHO, 2014). Within low- and middle-income countries, the highest estimated rates of homicide occur in the Americas, 28.5 per 100,000 population, with a lifetime risk of becoming a homicide victim of about 1 in 85 for men and 1 in 280 for women.

There is little current data that estimates the percentage of severely mentally ill individuals who become violent. In the United States, a 1988 Department of Justice study reported that individuals with a history of mental illness (excluding drug or alcohol use) were responsible for 4.3% of homicides (897 out of 20,860). In instances in which the homicide occurred among family members, the percentage was much higher—for example, in 25% of cases in which an individual killed their parent, that individual was mentally ill (Dawson and Langan, 1994). Studies of violence among seriously mentally ill individuals have been reported in the

DOI: 10.4324/9781003137597-4

United States since 1990, indicating that 5–10% of such individuals commit acts of serious violence each year.

However, studies have also shown the importance of treatment to reduce this violence (Torrey, 2006). Therefore, during the psychiatric evaluation, identifying a client who is at risk for violent behaviors can assist the advanced psychiatric mental health nurse (APMHN) to prepare specific interventions to reduce that client's subjective distress, thereby diminishing the overall risk of harm and safeguarding clients, staff, and others with whom the client comes in contact from potentially violent behavior. This chapter will discuss how the APMHN can identify violent clients and conduct an appropriate assessment of them, as it is among the most critical tasks in psychiatry.

Section 1: Assessment of Suicidal Clients

Suicide assessment is an essential first step in helping APMHNs estimate a client's risk for suicide. After that assessment has been conducted, a determination can be made as to an appropriate treatment setting, and an individualized treatment plan can be formulated that addresses specific modifiable risk factors, including any need for heightened observation. A suicide assessment protocol is composed of the following steps: (1) gathering information related to a client's risk and protective factors, and the warning signs for suicide; (2) gathering information related to the client's suicidal ideation, planning, behaviors, desire, and intent; and (3) the clinical decision-making that is subsequently applied to create a formulation of risk.

Inquiring about suicidal thoughts during the initial psychiatric evaluation may improve the identification of clients who are at increased risk of suicide, and specific interventions may be able to reduce the client's subjective distress and overall risk of self-injury or death. However, when communicating with the client, it is important to remember that simply asking about suicidal ideas or other elements of the assessment will not ensure that accurate or complete information is received. For example, during the initial evaluation, the client may appear to be cooperative with the assessment and forthcoming with answers to questions; however, if the client appears to be sullen, guarded, irritable, or agitated, the APMHN may find the information limited to behavioral observations.

The APMHN should consider several elements when assessing a client's risk of suicide:

1. There is no evidence that risk of suicide is increased by asking a client directly about current suicidal ideas, plans, and/or intents.
2. If a client appears to minimize the severity of suicidal behaviors, or if the clinical presentation seems inconsistent with an initial denial of suicidal thoughts, additional questioning of the client or of significant others may be indicated.
3. Cultural factors are important to consider when framing questions, since issues such as shame, guilt, or humiliation can be culturally mediated and

influence a client's risk of or willingness to discuss suicidal thoughts or suicide plans.

4. Factors involving the interviewing clinician, such as time pressures, interviewing style, and preconceived notions about suicide, can influence the ability to conduct an accurate assessment.

5. Clients with an intellectual disability or a neurocognitive disorder may have difficulty understanding questions as initially posed, and flexibility may be needed to reframe questions in a clearer manner.

6. Using open-ended questions rather than closed ones is more conducive to capturing the nuances and narrative of the client's concerns, with follow-up questioning as needed to hone in on additional details.

7. No study has demonstrated which population-based risk factors or combinations of them can accurately predict which clients will die by suicide. Accordingly, estimation of an individual client's risk for suicide is ultimately a matter of clinician judgment, which requires synthesizing the available information and deciding how to weigh the contributions of multiple factors.

8. In synthesizing and documenting information gained from the initial evaluation, the APMHN should focus primarily on estimating the patient's immediate suicide risk, while also taking into account longer-term contributors to risk that may need to be considered in treatment planning.

(Adapted from American Psychiatric Association [APA], 2016)

A. **Risk factors associated with suicide in the United States**

1. **Gender:**
   - Women attempt suicide four times more often than do men.
   - Men commit suicide three times more often than do women.
2. **Age:**
   - The suicide rate tends to increase with age, peaks after age 45 for men and after age 65 for women.
   - The most rapid increase in suicide is currently among 15–24-year-old males.
3. **Race:**
   - Two out of every three suicides are committed by white males.
   - Suicide rates are higher than average for Native Americans and Inuits.
4. **Marital status:**
   - Single persons are twice as likely as married persons to attempt suicide.
   - Divorced, separated, or widowed persons are four to five times as likely as married persons to attempt suicide.
5. **Health status:**
   - Those with chronic physical illness, especially if associated with chronic pain or terminal illness, are at least twice as likely to report

suicidal behaviors or to complete suicide; it is of the utmost importance to target which risk factors contribute the most to increasing suicidality (Racine, 2018).

- Mental illnesses: 95% of all suicides occur in people suffering from a psychiatric disturbance.
- Depressive disorders: 50% of all persons who commit suicide are depressed.
- Panic disorder: Almost 20% of all clients diagnosed with panic disorder attempt suicide, and 1% commit suicide.
- Schizophrenia: Approximately 4,000 clients with schizophrenia commit suicide each year; approximately 10% of those who have prominent delusions and command hallucinations telling them to harm themselves are at increased risk.
- Personality disorders (PDs):

  - Borderline personality disorder is associated with a high rate of para-suicidal behavior, such as self-injury directed at the surface of the body to induce relief from a negative feeling.
  - Antisocial personality disorder: Approximately 5% of clients with this disorder commit suicide.

6. **Substance dependence:**
   - Alcohol dependence increases the risk of comorbid depressive disorders by two-thirds and consequently increases the risk of suicide.
   - Heroin and other forms of substance dependence increase the suicide rate by approximately 20 times that of the general population.
7. **Other risk factors:**
   - Unambiguous wish to die.
   - Sense of hopelessness.
   - Hoarding pills.
   - Access to lethal agents or firearms.
   - Previous suicide attempt(s).
   - Family history of suicide or depression.
   - Fantasies of reunion with deceased loved ones.
   - History of childhood physical or sexual abuse.
   - History of impulsive or aggressive behavior.

(Adapted from Sadock et al., 2019)

Risk factors for suicide can vary among individuals, such as revenge, shame, humiliation, delusional guilt, command hallucinations, wanting to gain attention or a reaction from others, escaping physical or psychological pain, loneliness, self-hatred, or a sense of being a burden, of not belonging, of feeling trapped, or of having no purpose. In contrast, protective factors from suicide can include religious beliefs, a sense of responsibility to children or others, strong social support, plans for the future, or a sense of purpose in life. Given the large number of possible factors that can affect the risk of suicide, the APMHN can neither review nor document all of them, but can provide an estimated level of suicide risk, including risk and/or protective factors. It may also be helpful to conceptualize the overall risk in terms of underlying nonmodifiable risk factors as well as more immediate precipitants that may contribute to acute risk but are more likely to be modifiable (APA, 2016).

B. **Sample questions for assessment of current and prior suicidal thoughts and behaviors**
   1. **Addressing the client's general suicidal ideas, plans, and intent, including active or passive thoughts of suicide or death:**
      - *Have you ever felt that life was not worth living?*
      - *Did you ever wish not to wake up from sleeping?*
      - *Is death something you have thought about recently?*
      - *Have things ever reached the point that you have thought about suicide?*
   2. **If the client reports current suicidal ideas, the following questions are warranted:**
      Client's intended course of action if current symptoms worsen.
      - *Question: Have you made any specific plan to end your life if you feel that things are not working out?*
      Access to suicide methods, including firearms.
      - *Question: Have you made any particular preparations, such as writing a note or a will, making financial arrangements, or purchasing a gun or weapon?*
      Client's possible motivations for suicide (e.g., attention or reaction from others, revenge, shame, humiliation, delusional guilt, command hallucinations).
      - *Question: What led up to your suicidal thoughts?*
      Reasons for living (e.g., sense of responsibility to children or others, religious beliefs).
      - *Question: What things in your life lead you to want to go on living?*
      Quality and strength of the therapeutic alliance.
      - *Question: What things in your life make you feel more hopeful about the future?*
   3. **Addressing the client's past history of suicidal ideas, plans, and attempts, including attempts that were aborted or interrupted, as well as prior intentional self-injury in which there was no suicide intent:**
      - *Was there a time in the past when you tried to end your life? And can you describe what happened?*
      - *What were the circumstances that led you to suicidal thoughts (e.g., divorce, loss of job or loved one, a serious health issue)?*
      - *How close did you come to acting on the suicidal thoughts?*
      - *What thoughts were you having beforehand that led up to the suicidal attempt?*

- *Was anyone present when you made the suicidal attempt?*
- *How did you feel afterward (e.g., relief or regret about being alive)?*
- *Did you receive treatment following your suicidal thought or attempt?*

4. **For individuals with psychosis, ask specifically about hallucinations and delusions:**
   - *Can you describe the voices (e.g., single versus multiple, male versus female, internal versus external, recognizable versus stranger)?*
   - *What do the voices say?*
   - *Have there been times when the voices told you to hurt or kill yourself?*
   - *Have you ever done what the voices asked you to do?*

(Adapted from Sadock et al., 2019).

C. **Interviewing techniques when assessing suicidal clients: Chronological Assessment of Suicide Events (CASE) approach**

The ultimate goal of the interviewing strategy is to help the clinician assess the client's actual suicidal intent by maximizing the validity of their stated and reflected intent while minimizing their withheld intent. The Chronological Assessment of Suicide Events (CASE) approach is a highly organized interviewing technique that has been positively received by mental health professionals and suicidologists, substance abuse counselors, primary care clinicians, clinicians in the correctional system, legal experts, military/ VA mental health professionals, and psychiatric residency directors (Shea, 2004). The CASE approach provides APMHNs with a practical framework for exploring and better understanding how to elicit suicidal ideation, behavior, desire, and intent in a client so that the APMHN can develop an individualized approach with which they feel comfortable and competent.

1. **Validity techniques of the CASE approach**

The CASE validity techniques emphasize the impact of the questions the APMHN asks and of how the APMHN asks them. Two validity techniques proven to be valuable are normalization and shame attenuation.

   a. **Normalization** is a process of normalizing a topic for the client, and is an unobtrusive method of raising the issue of suicide. For example, the APMHN might say, "Sometimes when people feel as much pain as you are feeling, they have thought of killing themselves. Has that happened to you?"

   b. **Shame attenuation** is based on the assumption that if a client answers positively to sensitive questions, such as about suicide attempts or thoughts, they are in essence admitting a failure and then feel shame. With shame attenuation, the client's own pain is used as the gateway to the topic of suicide to reduce the shame by discussing suicide openly and nonjudgmentally. The APMHN might ask, "Considering all of the pain you've been feeling in the past couple of weeks, I'm wondering if you have had any thoughts of killing yourself?"

Four cornerstones of these validity techniques are used to explore the extent of suicidal ideation:

a. **Behavioral incident:** Questions that ask for specific facts, behavioral details, or trains of thought. By asking about a series of behavioral incidents, the interviewer can sometimes help a patient to share thoughts and feelings honestly by re-creating, step by step, the unfolding of a potentially taboo topic, such as a suicidal attempt, thereby enabling the interviewer to get accurate information. The following are prototypes of typical behavioral incidents and related sample questions:

- Fact-finding behavioral incident sample questions:
- "How many pills did you take?"
- "Did you put the razor blade to your wrist?
- "How many bottles of pills did you actually store up?"
- "When you say that 'you tried to end it all,' what did you actually do?"
- Sequencing behavioral incident sample questions:
- "What did you do next?" or "What did your wife do then?"
- "What did your husband say right after he found out that you tried to hang yourself?"
- "Can you tell me what happened next?"

Clinical caveat: Behavioral incidents are excellent at uncovering hidden information, but are time-consuming. Therefore, using only this clinical approach can be impractical when the APMHN is pressured for sufficient time to do a full initial intake. With a potentially suicidal client, the APMHN must be selective as to when to employ behavioral incidents and when to employ other questioning techniques.

b. **Gentle assumption:** Gentle assumption can be used when the APMHN suspects that a client may be hesitant to discuss a suicidal behavior. With gentle assumption, the APMHN assumes that the potentially embarrassing or incriminating behavior is occurring and frames each question accordingly, in a gentle tone of voice. The following are prototypes of gentle assumption sample questions:

- What kinds of problems have you had at work?
- What other ways have you thought of killing yourself?

Clinical caveat: Gentle assumptions are powerful examples of leading questions and therefore must be used with care. They should not be used with clients who may feel intimidated by the APMHN or who are trying to provide what they think the APMHN wants to hear.

c. **Denial of the specific:** After a client has denied a generic question, it is surprising how asking a series of specific questions can jar the client's memory. This approach can also be effective as it appears to be harder to falsely deny a specific as opposed to a generic question. The following are prototypes of denial of the specific sample questions:

- Have you ever thought of shooting yourself?
- Have you ever thought of overdosing?
- Have you ever thought of hanging yourself?

Clinical caveat: It is important for the APMHN to frame each denial of the specific as a separate question, pausing between each inquiry and waiting for the client's denial or admission before asking the next question. The clinician should avoid combining the inquiries into a single question, such as, "Have you ever thought of shooting yourself, overdosing, or hanging yourself?" A series of items combined in this way is called a "cannon question," and can frequently lead to invalid information, as clients generally only hear parts of them or respond to only one item in the string, often the last one.

    d. **Symptom amplification:** This technique is based on the observation that clients often minimize the frequency of their disturbing behaviors, such as the frequency with which they cut their wrists or think about overdosing on pills. In such a situation, symptom amplification is used in an effort to determine the frequency of a particular behavior without creating a confrontational atmosphere. For a question to be viewed as symptom amplification, the APMHN must suggest a specific number of times, set high, that a client practices a behavior. It therefore should only be used if the APMHN suspects that the client is about to minimize, not maximize, as clients who do the latter tend to seek attention from others. The following is a prototype of a symptom amplification sample question:

- "On the days when your thoughts of suicide are most intense, how much of your time do you spend thinking about killing yourself ... 70% of your waking hours, 80%, 90%?"

Clinical caveat: It is important not to set the upper limit at such a high number that it seems absurd or creates the appearance that the APMHN does not know what they are talking about.

2. **Sequence of the CASE approach**

In the CASE approach, the clinician sequentially explores the following four chronological steps:

Step 1: Presenting suicide events (within the past 48 hours).

Step 2: Recent suicide events (within the preceding 2 months).

Step 3: Past suicide events (from 2 months ago and further back in time).

Step 4: Immediate suicide events (suicidal feelings, ideation, and intent that arise during the interview itself).

The term "suicide events" includes any of the following: death wishes, suicidal feelings and thoughts, planning, behaviors, desire, and intent.

Step 1: Exploration of presenting suicide events

Whether the client spontaneously raises the topic of suicide or the APMHN sensitively uncovers it with techniques such as normalization or shame attenuation, suicidal events are viewed as "presenting suicide events" if they occurred within the last 48 hours. If a client presents with such current suicidal behavior or with pressing suicidal ideation, it becomes critical to understand the severity of the attempt or ideation, as the APMHN's formulation of the client's immediate risk will determine the urgency of recommended follow-up, whether from an emergency department (ED) or from a crisis hotline.

The exploration of presenting suicide events can be summarized as follows:

1. The APMHN begins with a question, such as, "It sounds like last night was a very difficult time. It will help me to understand exactly what you experienced if you can sort of walk me through what happened step by step."
2. As the client begins to describe the unfolding suicide attempt, to maximize validity the APMHN can use one or two anchor questions, which aim to anchor the client into a specific memory, as opposed to recalling a collection of nebulous feelings. Such a refined focus will often bring forth more valid information as the episode becomes both more real and more vivid to the client. For example, for a client with a suicide event involving a gun, the APMHN could ask anchor questions such as, "When did you take the gun out?" and "Where were you sitting when you had the gun out?"

    The APMHN then proceeds to use a series of behavioral incident questions, making it easy to picture the unfolding events—the "verbal videotape." For example, if the APMHN uses a mix of fact-finding and sequencing behavioral incident questions with a client who took some actions with a gun, the series may look something like the following:

"Do you have a gun in the house?"
"Have you ever gotten the gun out with the thought of using it to kill yourself?"
"When did you do this?"
"Where were you sitting when you had the gun out?"
"Did you load the gun?"
"What did you do next?" (sequencing behavioral incident)
"Did you put the gun up to your body or your head?"
"Did you take the safety off or load the chamber?"
"How long did you hold the gun there?"
"What thoughts were going through your mind then?"
"What did you do then?" (sequencing behavioral incident)
"What stopped you from pulling the trigger?"

Step 2: Exploration of recent suicide events

Often, the APMHN can elicit the client's thoughts about recent suicide events—that is, events that occurred within the preceding 2 months—once presenting suicide events have been explored. A gentle assumption is used to look for a second suicide attempt or method by asking, for example, "What other ways have you thought of killing yourself?" This type of question can elicit more information from the client, as it cannot simply be answered yes or no. If the same plan was recently contemplated or if a second method is uncovered, sequential behavioral incident questions are used to create another verbal videotape. After establishing the list of methods considered by the client and the extent of action taken for each method, the APMHN hones in on the frequency, duration, and intensity of the suicidal ideation by using symptom amplification. For example,

1. "Over the past 2 months, during the days when you were most thinking about killing yourself, how much time did you spend thinking about it … 70% of your waking hours, 80%? 90%?"

Step 3: Exploration of past suicide events

What past suicidal history—that is, suicide events from 2 months ago and further back in time—is important to gather? For clinical efficacy, and given that the APMHN will likely have a limited amount of time for the initial assessment, only information that could potentially change the clinical triage and any decisions about client follow-up should be sought. Thus, the following questions are worth investigating:

1. What is the most serious past suicide attempt? (Is the current ideation focused on the same method? Does the client view the current stressors and options in the same light as during the most dangerous past attempt?)
2. Are the current triggers and the client's current psychopathological state similar to when the most serious attempts were made? (The client may be prone to suicide following the break-up of relationships or during episodes of acute intoxication, intense anxiety, or psychosis.)
3. What is the approximate number of past gestures and attempts? (Large numbers can point to issues of manipulation, making the APMHN less concerned, or to the possibility that the patient has truly exhausted all hope, making the APMHN more concerned. In either case, it is important to know.)
4. When was the most recent attempt outside of the 2 months explored in Step 2? (There could have been a significant attempt within the past 6 months that may signal the need for more immediate concern.)

Step 4: Exploration of immediate suicide events

Here, the interviewer focuses on, "What is this client's suicidal intent right now?" The APMHN explores any suicidal ideation, intent, and plan that the client may be experiencing during the interview itself and also inquires whether the client thinks they are likely to have further thoughts of suicide after leaving the office, ED, or inpatient unit, or gets off the phone following a crisis call, depending on where the assessment is taking place. The region of immediate events also includes any appropriate safety planning. The focus of the exploration of immediate events is thus on the present and future.

A sound starting place is the question, "Right now, are you having any thoughts about wanting to kill yourself?" From this inquiry, a variety of questions can be used to further explore the client's desire to die, such as:

- "How would you describe how bad the pain is for you in your divorce right now, ranging from 'It's sort of tough, but I can handle it okay' to 'If it doesn't let up, I don't know if I can go on?'"
- "In the upcoming week, how will you handle your pain if it worsens?"

Questions such as the following can help delineate intent:

- "I realize that you can't know for sure, but what is your best guess as to how likely it is that you will try to kill yourself during the next week, ranging from highly unlikely to very likely?"
- "What keeps you from killing yourself?"

It is important to explore the client's current level of hopelessness and to assess whether the client is making productive plans for the future or is amenable to preparing concrete plans for dealing with current problems and stresses. Questions such as the following may be asked:

- "How does the future look to you?"
- "Do you feel hopeful about the future?"
- "What things would make you feel more or less hopeful about the future?"
- "What things in your life make you want to go on living?"

(Adapted from Shea, 1998, 2002, 2009)

It is important to note that while the CASE approach is a flexible interview strategy, it is devoted solely to the elicitation of suicidal events and is therefore always employed within the context of some other clinical interview, such as an initial psychiatric assessment. In addition, the CASE approach is not a method of uncovering risk/protective factors for suicide; rather, such vital information should be gathered during a full mental status examination of, for example, the client's history of substance use, the presence and intensity of the client's anxiety/agitation, and/or the presence of psychosis.

Section 2: Assessment of Other-Directed Violence, including Aggressive Behaviors and Homicide

The criminological and psychiatric literature suggests that risk factors for other-directed violence, including homicide, are in some respects different for people with mental disorders than for the general population (Buchanan et al., 2012). The mental disorders most commonly associated with aggressive behaviors leading to other-directed violence are paranoia, command hallucination, and substance intoxication. Diagnoses that tend to show aggressive behaviors are personality disorders (i.e., borderline and antisocial PDs), which are characterized by rage and poor impulse control, and cognitive disorders (typically those associated with frontal and temporal lobe involvement) (Sadock et al., 2019). Therefore, it is essential that the APMHN evaluate a client's risk for other-directed violence during the initial psychiatric evaluation. (*Please note that the term "violence" is commonly used in the literature to refer to "other-directed violence," and therefore will be used in that way for the rest of this section.*)

Evaluating such risk in a client is ultimately a matter of clinician judgment that requires synthesizing the available information and deciding how to weigh the contributions of multiple factors, including those that may encourage the client to violently act on aggressive ideas as well as those that may discourage them from doing so. This clinical decision-making process and a discussion of the factors that are judged to influence the client's risk of aggressive and violent behavior should be included in the clinical documentation, typically in a brief paragraph. Distinctions between modifiable risk factors (e.g., alcohol or substance use, psychosis) that could be reduced by treatment or other interventions, and static, nonmodifiable risk factors (e.g., age, sex, clinical history) are also important to note in assessing and documenting risk and arriving at a plan for addressing it (APA, 2016).

Risk Factors for Aggressive and Violent Behaviors

1. **Nonmodifiable risk factors:**
   - Sociodemographic:
     - Young age (late teens or early 20s).
     - Male.
   - Personal history:
     - History of aggressive and violent behaviors, impulsivity, in similar circumstances.
     - Recent act(s) of violence/destruction of property.
     - History of being physically abused in childhood.
     - History of being exposed to violent behaviors of other family members.
2. **Modifiable risk factors:**
   - Presence of symptoms of psychiatric disorders:
     - Substance use: Alcohol or stimulant intoxication.
     - PDs: Antisocial PD, borderline PD.
     - Psychosis: Symptoms of paranoid delusions, command hallucinations.
     - Psychiatric disorders secondary to a general medical condition: Dementia, delirium.
     - Intermittent explosive disorder.

- Environment:
  - Weapons available: Remove by either client's family member or legal authority.
  - Intended victim(s) picked out: Apply the Tarasoff duty to protect following the requirements of the local jurisdiction.

3. **Additional risk factors to be considered in EDs and inpatient units:**
   - Aggressive attributional style (hostile, suspicious, or believing others intend harm).
   - Command hallucinations to harm others.
   - Poor therapeutic alliance has been implicated.
   - Some paraphilias are risk factors for sexual offending.

The APA (2016) recommends that the initial psychiatric evaluation of a client include an assessment of current and past aggressive or psychotic ideas, including thoughts of physical or sexual aggression or homicide. Skillful clinicians assessing the possibility of a client's dangerous behavior formulate and test a series of clinical hypotheses to define any patterns of violence in the individual's history. Once defined, these patterns can be utilized to explain and predict a client's potential for violence. The APA (2016) proposes the following guidelines of risk assessment for aggressive/violent behaviors.

Guidelines of Risk Assessment for Aggressive/Violent Behaviors

1. **The initial psychiatric evaluation of a client includes assessing:**
   - Current and prior aggressive or psychotic ideas, including thoughts of physical or sexual aggression or homicide (e.g., command hallucinations).
   - Past aggressive/violent behaviors (e.g., homicide, domestic or workplace violence, other physically or sexually aggressive threats or acts), as this is the most robust statistical indicator of further violence.
   - Consequences of past aggressive behaviors leading to legal or disciplinary actions, psychiatric hospitalization, and/or ED visits.
   - History of violent behaviors in biological relatives.
   - Current or recent substance use disorder or change in use of alcohol or other substances.
   - Presence of psychosocial stressors.
   - Exposure to violence or aggressive behavior, including combat exposure or childhood abuse.
   - Past or current neurological or neurocognitive disorders or symptoms.
2. **When it is determined during an initial psychiatric evaluation that the client has aggressive ideas, the APA recommends assessing:**
   - Impulsivity, including anger management issues.
   - Access to firearms.

- Specific individuals or groups toward whom homicidal or aggressive ideas or behaviors have been directed in the past or at present.
- History of violent behaviors in biological relatives.

3. **The clinician who conducts the initial psychiatric evaluation should document an estimation of risk of aggressive behavior (including homicide), including factors influencing risk.**

Inquiring during the initial psychiatric evaluation about aggressive and violent behaviors and thoughts, as well as about related risk or protective factors, may improve the identification of clients who are at increased risk of violent behaviors. If aggressive and violent thoughts or other modifiable risk factors are found, specific interventions may be able to reduce the client's subjective distress and diminish the overall risk of harm by determining an appropriate treatment setting and formulating an individualized treatment plan that may include heightened observation or may target specific modifiable risk factors. However, there is no evidence that assessing any of these factors or utilizing specific violence rating scales can predict violence in an individual. Despite these limitations, there is consensus by experts that the benefits of assessing the factors described in the above guidelines in an initial psychiatric evaluation clearly outweigh the potential harms, including unclear costs.

(Modified guideline statements for assessment of risk for aggressive behaviors, APA, 2016)

Management of Aggressive, Violent, or Homicidal Clients during the Psychiatric Evaluation

Managing aggressive, violent, or homicidal clients in psychiatric practice involves a range of activities, from prescribing appropriate treatment to ensuring a safe environment.

1. **The APMHN should always protect self:**
   - Assume that violence and homicide are always a possibility.
   - Never interview an armed client (the client should always surrender a weapon or potential weapon to secure personnel).
   - Know as much as possible about the client before the interview.
   - Never interview a potentially violent client alone or in an office with the door closed.
   - Remove neckties, necklaces, and other articles of clothing or jewelry that the client can grab or pull.
   - Stay within sight of other staff members.
   - Keep at least an arm's length away from any potentially violent client.
   - Always leave a route of rapid escape in case the client attacks you.
   - Never turn your back on the client.
2. **Observation of signs of impending violence and homicide:**
   - Psychomotor agitation.
   - Recent violent acts against people or property.

- Clenched teeth and fists, verbal threats.
- Possession of weapons or of objects potentially usable as weapons.
- Drug or alcohol intoxication.
- Paranoid delusions and/or command hallucinations.
3. **Provide a nonstimulating environment.**
4. **Explore possible psychosocial interventions to reduce the risk of violence and homicide (e.g., if violence is related to a specific situation or person, try to separate the client from that situation or person).**
5. **Intended victims must be warned of the continued possibility of danger (e.g., if the client is not hospitalized).**

(Adapted from Sadock et al., 2019)

There are different approaches to violence risk assessment, such as clinical assessment and anamnestic assessment. In general, a mental health clinician conducts clinical risk assessment of violence by gathering information related to a potential risk, including history, which is then processed by the clinician to offer their clinical impressions and judgments. It is a relatively unstructured approach by which the mental health clinician gathers whatever information they believe to be relevant to the assessment and prediction task, and processes it in whatever way they consider appropriate. Anamnestic risk assessment is a specific type of clinical assessment whereby the examiner attempts to identify violence risk factors through a detailed examination of the individual's history of violent and threatening behavior. Through a clinical interview, review of third-party information (e.g., arrest reports, hospital accounts, reports of significant others), and perhaps psychological or other types of testing, the examining clinician tries to identify themes or commonalities across violence episodes that can be used to articulate risk or protective factors specific to the individual.

Violence Screening Sample Questions

1. **Screening Questions during General Clinical Assessment:**
   - What kinds of things make you mad? What do you do when you get mad?
   - What is your temper like? What kinds of things can make you lose your temper?
   - What is the most violent thing you have ever done and how did it happen?
   - What is the closest you have ever come to being violent?
   - Have you ever used a weapon in a fight or to hurt someone?
   - What would have to happen for you to get so mad or angry that you would hurt someone?
   - Do you own weapons like guns or knives? Where are they now?
2. **Anamnestic Violence Risk Analysis: Detailed Questions Related to Specific Incidents:**
   - What kind(s) of harm occurred?
   - Who were the victims(s) and/or targets?

- In what setting or environment did the altercation(s) take place?
- What do you think caused the violence?
- What were you thinking before the altercation(s)?
- What were you thinking during the altercation(s)?
- What were you thinking after the altercations(s)?
- How were you feeling before the altercation(s)?
- How were you feeling during the altercation(s)?
- How were you feeling after the altercation(s)?
- Were you using alcohol or other drugs at or around the time of the altercation(s)?
- Was the client experiencing psychotic symptoms, such as threat/control-override (TCO) symptoms, at the time of the altercation? (A question asked to a third-party informant to gather information.)
- Were you taking psychoactive medication at the time of the incident?
- Can patterns or commonalities across this and other episodes be identified?

(Adapted from Borum et al., 1996)

In the process of violence risk assessment, APMHNs will find that they must communicate their impressions, formulations, and recommendations to various third parties, either informally (e.g., in discussions with the client or significant others) or formally (e.g., in the context of a civil commitment proceeding or to the treatment team). At least in more formal contexts, care should be taken that impressions of the risk of violence and any recommended responses and interventions are communicated clearly, and that any limitations of their opinions are made known (Otto, 2000).

References

American Psychiatric Association (APA). (2016). *Practice guidelines for the psychiatric evaluation of adults* (3rd ed.). American Psychiatric Association. https://doi.org/10.1176/appi.pn.2015.8a5

Borum, R., Swartz, M., & Swanson, J. (1996). Assessing and managing violence risk in clinical practice. *Journal of Practical Psychiatry and Behavioral Health, 2*, 205–215.

Buchanan, A., Binder, R., Norko, M., & Swartz, M. (2012). Resource document on psychiatric violence risk assessment. *The American Journal of Psychiatry, 169*(3), 340. https://doi.org/10.1176/appi.ajp.2012.169.3.340

Dawson, J. M., & Langan, P. A. (1994). *Murder in families.* Bureau of Justice Statistics, U.S. Department of Justice. www.mentalillnesspolicy.org/consequences/1000-hom

Otto, R. K. (2000). Assessing and managing violence risk in outpatient settings. *Journal of Clinical Psychology, 56*(10), 1239–1262.

Racine, M. (2018). Chronic pain and suicide risk: A comprehensive review. *Progress in Neuro-psychopharmacology and Biological Psychiatry, 87*, 269–280. https://doi: 10.1016/j

Sadock, B., Ahmad, S., & Sadock, V. (2019). *Kaplan & Sadock's pocket handbook of clinical psychiatry* (6th ed.). Wolters Kluwer.

Shea, S. C. (1998). The chronological assessment of suicide events: A practical interviewing strategy for eliciting suicidal ideation. *Journal of Clinical Psychiatry, 59*(suppl 20), 58–72.

Shea, S. C. (2002). *The practical art of suicide assessment: A guide for mental health professionals and substance abuse counselors.* Wiley.

Shea, S. C. (2004). The delicate art of eliciting suicidal ideation. *Psychiatric Annals, 34,* 385–400.

Shea, S. C. (2009). Suicide assessment: Part 2: Uncovering suicidal intent using the chronological assessment of suicide events (CASE Approach). *Psychiatric Times.* www.psychiatrictimes.com/suicide/suicide-assessment-part-2-uncovering-suicidal -intentusing-case-approach

Torrey, E. F. (2006). Violence and schizophrenia. *Schizophrenia Research, 88*(1–3), 3–4. https://doi.org/10.1016/j.schres.2006.09.010

World Health Organization (WHO). (2014, January). *Global status report on violence prevention 2014.* World Health Organization. www.medicinecontact.com/world-report -on-violence-and-prevention-world-health-organization

World Health Organization. (2019). *Suicide in the world: Global health estimates.* World Health Organization. https://apps.who.int/iris/handle/10665/326948

4 Practice Guidelines for Cultural Assessments

The term "culture" refers to a large and diverse set of mostly intangible aspects of social life: the values, beliefs, systems of language, communication, and practices that people share and that can be used to define them as a collective (Cole, 2020). It is important that advanced psychiatric mental health nurses (APMHNs) be aware that individuals present for psychiatric assessment from a wide range of cultural backgrounds, and that factors such as age, ethnicity, gender, race, religion, and sexual orientation can shape a client's personal and cultural identity, as well as influence their beliefs about, and communications with, mental health professionals, who, for example, the client may view as authority figures. In addition, individuals from different backgrounds may differ in their understanding and views of mental illness, as well as in their preferences for psychiatric treatment, particularly given cross-cultural differences in the possible stigma attached to psychiatric disorders (Abdullah & Brown, 2011; Angermeyer & Dietrich, 2006; Jimenez et al., 2012; Lim, 2015).

Cultural differences also can be associated with disparities in medical care and health outcomes (Gone & Trimble, 2012; Hall-Lipsy & Chisholm-Burns, 2010; Thomas et al., 2011). Gone and Trimble (2012) report that American Indians and Alaska Natives suffer from specific mental health disparities, including disproportionately high rates of substance abuse, post-traumatic stress, youth behavior problems, and suicide. In their literature review investigating whether race, ethnicity, or sex are associated with disparities in medication treatment, Hall-Lipsy and Chisholm-Burns (2010) found significant disparities among racial/ethnic minorities and women. With the aim of eliminating health disparities, achieving health equity has been a goal of Healthy People 2030. However, despite the improvement in the health status of the US population as a whole, racial/ethnic minorities continue to lag behind whites, with a quality of life diminished by illness from preventable chronic diseases and a life span cut short by premature death (Thomas et al., 2011). Healthy People 2030 describes a vision for all people in the United States to achieve their full potential for health and well-being across the life span, which will benefit society as a whole. Gaining such benefits requires eliminating health disparities, achieving health equity, attaining health literacy, and strengthening physical, social, and economic environments (Pronk et al., 2021).

DOI: 10.4324/9781003137597-5

Consequently, the relevance of cultural factors to both diagnosis and treatment strongly suggests the potential benefits of identifying each client's cultural beliefs during the initial psychiatric evaluation, as such beliefs can influence the therapeutic alliance, promote diagnostic accuracy, and enable appropriate treatment planning (American Psychiatric Association [APA], 2013). The APA (2013) recommends three guidelines for doing so.

Guideline 1: Assess the client's need for an interpreter

For many clients, the need for an interpreter and the appropriateness of different interpreter options should be identified during the initial visit. Although language-concordant clinicians or trained in-person interpreters have typically been used, other ways for accessing professional interpreters are increasingly available, such as telephonic- and video-based options, as well as remote interpreting services. Some clients who are deaf or hard of hearing may prefer to communicate through an in-person or video-based sign language interpreter, whereas others may prefer to communicate through other approaches, such as lip reading, face-to-face keyboards, and writing.

Guideline 2: Assess cultural factors related to the client's social environment

There is substantial heterogeneity as to how clients gain support or feel estranged from cultural networks, making it important to explore the client's views and feelings. When present, social networks (e.g., religious affiliations, tribal supports, military command structure) within a client's culture can help to strengthen their social ties and supports. For example, in many cultures, families are an important source of support during times of illness, and in some cultures, treatment decisions are made by family members rather than by the individual client.

Guideline 3: Assess the client's personal/cultural beliefs and cultural explanations of psychiatric illness

Individuals from a specific cultural group will have a wide range of beliefs. Some clients may use culturally specific treatments, such as medications, supplements, health practices, and consultations with culturally specific healers. Family members or members of a client's cultural group may also be helpful in explaining the client's belief systems, as well as whether their current beliefs and behaviors are or are not in keeping with those of the client's cultural group. Typical examples are spiritual beliefs that are not part of an organized religion, or cultural or religious rituals.

Lim (2015) recommends that healthcare providers use the *Diagnostic and Statistical Manual of Mental Disorders* (DSM-5) (APA, 2013), Cultural Formulation Interview (CFI) as a cultural assessment instrument to learn about cultures that are represented among their clients, as well as to improve their ability to assess cultural factors that are relevant to diagnosis and treatment. The DSM-5 presents two versions of the CFI: (1) the CFI—Client Version, with 16 questions; and (2) the CFI—Informant Version, with 17 questions. The questions for each version are listed below for APMHNs to review so that they can use the ones they deem most relevant during the initial psychiatric evaluation. Detailed information about and instructions for each of these questions, as well as additional extended questions, can be found in the DSM-5 (APA, 2013).

    I. **The CFI—Client Version** includes four assessment domains and a total of 16 questions.

Domain 1: Cultural Definition of the Problem

1. What brings you here today? (Problem identification)
2. Sometimes people have different ways of describing their problem to their family, friends, or others in their community. How would you describe your problem to them? (Description of problem)
3. What troubles you most about your problem? (Consequences of problem)

Domain 2: Cultural Perceptions of Cause, Context, and Support

4. Why do you think this is happening to you? What troubles do you think are the causes of your problem? (Cause)
5. What do your family, friends, or others in your community think is causing your problem? (Cause)
6. Are there any kinds of supports that make your problem better, such as support from family, friends, or others? (Supports)
7. Are there any kinds of stresses that make your problem worse, such as difficulties with money or family problems? (Stressors)
8. For you, what are the most important aspects of your background or identity? (Role of cultural identity)
9. Are there any aspects of your background or identity that you believe make a difference to your problem? (Role of cultural identity)
10. Are there any aspects of your background or identity that are causing other concerns or difficulties for you? (Role of cultural identity)

Domain 3: Cultural Factors Affecting Self-Coping and Past Help Seeking

11. Sometimes people have various ways of dealing with problems like yours. What have you done on your own to cope with your problem? (Self-coping)
12. Often people look for help from many different sources, including different kinds of doctors, helpers, or healers. In the past, what kinds of treatment, help, advice, or healing have you sought for you problem? (Past help seeking)
13. Has anything prevented you from getting the help you need? (Barriers)

14. What kinds of help do you think would be most useful to you at this time for your problem? (Useful self-coping skills)
15. Are there other kinds of help that your family, friends, or other people have suggested that you believe would be helpful for you now? (External help)

Domain 4: Clinician–Client Relationship

16. Sometimes doctors and patients misunderstand each other because they come from different backgrounds or have different expectations. Have you been concerned about this kind of problem and is there anything we can do to provide you with the care you need? (Relationship)

II. **The CFI—Informant Version** includes five assessment domains, and a total of 17 questions. It is used to collect collateral information from a client's family, friends, or significant others who are familiar with the client's current issues and life circumstances. This version can be used to obtain information supplemental to that obtained during the CFI—Client Version or if the client is not able to provide information themselves.

Introduction for the Informant (client is assumed to be female and the informant's close friend):

"I would like to understand the problems that brought your friend here so that I can help you and her more effectively. Knowing more about your experiences and thoughts will help me to do that, so I will ask you some questions about what has happened and how you and she are dealing with it. I want you to know that there are no right or wrong answers."

Domain 1: Relationship with the Client

1. How would you describe your relationship with her? (Description of relationship)

Domain 2: Cultural Definition of the Problem

2. What brings your friend here today? (Problem identification)
3. Sometimes people have different ways of describing the problem to family, friends, or others in their community. How would you describe her problem to them? (Description of problem)
4. What troubles you most about her problem? (Consequences of problem)

Domain 3: Cultural Perceptions of Cause, Context, and Support

5. Why do you think this is happening to her? And what do you think are the causes of her problem? (Cause)

6. What do her family, other friends, or others in the community think is causing her problem? (Cause)
7. Are there any kinds of supports that make her problem better, such as from family, friends, or others? (Supports)
8. Are there any kinds of stresses that make her problem worse, such as difficulties with money or family problems? (Stressors)
9. For you, what are the most important aspects of her background or identity? (Role of cultural identity)
10. Are there any aspects of her background or identity that make a difference to her problem? (Role of cultural identity)
11. Are there any aspects of her background or identity that are causing other concerns or difficulties for her? (Role of cultural identity)

Domain 4: Cultural Factors Affecting Self-Coping and Past Help Seeking

12. Sometimes people have various ways of dealing with problems like hers. What has she done on her own to cope with her problem? (Self-coping)
13. Often people also look for help from many different sources, such as different kinds of doctors, helpers, or healers. In the past, what kinds of treatment, help, advice, or healing has she sought for her problem? (Past help seeking)
14. Has anything prevented her from getting the help she needs? (Barriers)

Domain 5: Cultural Factors Affecting Current Help Seeking

15. What kinds of help do you believe would be most useful to her at this time for her problem? (Perceived needs)
16. Are there other kinds of help that her family, friends, or other people have suggested that you believe would be helpful for her now? (Perceived expectation)
17. Have you been concerned about doctors and patients misunderstanding each other because they come from different backgrounds? And is there anything that we can do to provide her with the care she needs? (Clinician–client relationship)

(Adapted from DSM-5, APA, 2013)

References

Abdullah, T., & Brown, T. L. (2011). Mental illness stigma and ethnocultural beliefs, values, and norms: An integrative review. *Clinical Psychology Review, 31*(6), 934–948.

American Psychiatric Association (APA). (2013). *Diagnostic and statistical manual of mental disorders (DSM-5)* (5th ed., text rev.). Author.

Angermeyer, M. C., & Dietrich, S. (2006). Public beliefs about and attitudes towards people with mental illness: A review of population studies. *Acta Psychiatrica Scandinavica, 113*(3), 163–179.

Cole, N. L. (2020, August). So what is culture, exactly? *ThoughtCo.* www.thoughtco.com› culture-definition-4135409

Gone, J. P., & Trimble, J. E. (2012). American Indian and Alaska Native mental health: Diverse perspectives on enduring disparities. *Annual Review of Clinical Psychology, 8*, 131–160.

Hall-Lipsy, E. A., & Chisholm-Burns, M. A. (2010). Pharmacotherapeutic disparities: Racial, ethnic, and sex variations in medication treatment. *American Journal of Health: System Pharmacy, 67*(6), 462–468. http://doi: 10.2146/ajhp090161. PMID: 20208053

Jimenez, D. E., Bartels, S. J., Cardenas, V., Daliwal, S. S., & Alegría, M. (2012). Cultural beliefs and mental health treatment preferences of ethnically diverse older adult consumers in primary care. *American Journal of Geriatric Psychiatry, 20*(6), 533–542.

Lim, R. F. (2015). *Clinical manual of cultural psychiatry* (2nd ed.). American Psychiatric Publishing.

Pronk, N., Kleinman, D. V., Goekler, S. F., Ochiai, E., Blakey, C., & Brewer, K. H. (2021). Promoting health and well-being in Healthy People 2030. *Journal of Public Health Management and Practice, 27*(Suppl 6), S242–S248. https://doi.org/10.1097/PHH .0000000000001254

Thomas, S. B., Quinn, S. C., Butler, J., Fryer, C. S., & Garza, M. A. (2011). Toward a fourth generation of disparities research to achieve health equity. *Annual Review of Public Health, 32*, 399–416. https://doi.org/10.1146/annurev-publhealth-031210-101136

Index

Page numbers in **bold** indicate a table on the corresponding page

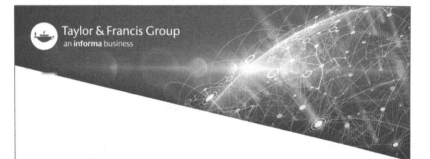

Printed in the United States
by Baker & Taylor Publisher Services